Unraveling the Origins:
Exploring 101 Triggers of Cancer

Table of Contents

INTRODUCTION 1

CHAPTER 1: WHAT IS CANCER? 2
    Free Radicals 2
    Cancer Treatment 3
    Cancer Classification 5
    1. Stage 0 (Carcinoma in Situ) 5
    2. Stage I (Early Stage) 5
    3. Stage II and III (Regional Spread) 5
    4. Stage IV (Distant Spread) 6
    Summary of the TNM System: 6

CHAPTER 2: A BRIEF HISTORY OF CANCER 7

CHAPTER 3: WHAT IS A CARCINOGEN? 9

CHAPTER 4. THE COST OF CANCER 12

CHAPTER 5: CANCER STATISTICS 14

CHAPTER 6: CANCER RESEARCH REPORTS 16

CHAPTER 7: ANIMAL TESTING 18

CHAPTER 8: CHEMICALS AND TOXICITY 21

CHAPTER 9: MY TOXICITY REPORT 23

CHAPTER 10: WE KNOW THE CAUSE — YET WE DO LITTLE FOR PREVENTION 27

CHAPTER 11: A TALE OF TWO CONSPIRACIES 30
    Big Tobacco 30
    Big Pharma 31

CHAPTER 12: LAWS AND CANCER WARNINGS 34
    United States: 34
    European Union: 36
    Canada: 36
    Australia: 36
    International: 36

CHAPTER 13: CANCER TRIGGERS 37

Trigger 1/101 – Tobacco Smoke 37
Trigger 2/101 – Formaldehyde 40
Trigger 3/101 – Asbestos 42
Trigger 4/101 – Haloacetic Acids 44
Trigger 5/101 – Dioxins... 46
Trigger 6/101 – Ultraviolet (UV) radiation... 48
Trigger 7/101 – Ionizing Radiation (X-rays, gamma rays) 49
Trigger 8/101 – Alcoholic Beverages 51
Trigger 9/101 – Nitrosamines... 53
Trigger 10/101 – Vinyl Chloride 55
Trigger 11/101 – Human Papillomavirus (HPV) 57
Trigger 12/101 – Hepatitis B Virus 59
Trigger 13/101 – Helicobacter Pylori 61
Trigger 14/101 – Aflatoxins 63
Trigger 15/101 – Benzidine 65
Trigger 16/101 – Cadmium (Smelting) 67
Trigger 17/101 – Chromium Hexavalent 69
Trigger 18/101 – Ethylene Oxide 71
Trigger 19/101 – Lead 72
Trigger 20/101 – Polycyclic Aromatic Hydrocarbon 75
Trigger 21/101 – Radon 77
Trigger 22/101 – Anabolic Steroids 79
Trigger 23/101 – Aristolochic Acids 83
Trigger 24/101 – Coal Tar 85
Trigger 25/101 – Secondhand Tobacco Smoke 86
Trigger 26/101 – Tamoxifen 89
Trigger 27/101 – 4-Aminobiphenyl... 91
Trigger 28/101 – Estrogen Replacement Therapy 93
Trigger 29/101 – MOOP Chemotherapy.. 95
Trigger 30/101 – Analgesic Mixtures Containing Phenacetin............ 96
Trigger 31/101 – Arsenic 100
Trigger 32/101 – Auramine 103
Trigger 33/101 – Benzo[a]pyrene... 105
Trigger 34/101 – Beryllium 107
Trigger 35/101 – Betel Quid 109
Trigger 36/101 – Bis(chloromethyl)ether and Chloromethyl Methyl Ether 111
Trigger 37/101 – 1,3-Butadiene.. 112
Trigger 38/101 – Captafol.. 114
Trigger 39/101 – Chlorambucil 115
Trigger 40/101 – Chlorinated paraffins 117
Trigger 41/101 – Semustine (MeCCNU) 120

- Trigger 42/101 – 2-Chloroethylvinyl Ether 122
- Trigger 43/101 – Chromium (VI) Compounds 124
- Trigger 44/101 – Cobalt Metal with Tungsten Carbide 125
- Trigger 45/101 – Combined Estrogen-Progestogen Menopausal Therapy (MHT) 128
- Trigger 46/101 – Contraceptives - Steroidal Estrogens 131
- Trigger 47/101 – Creosote 133
- Trigger 48/101 – Crystalline Silica 135
- Trigger 49/101 – Cyclamates 139
- Trigger 50/101 – Diethylstilbestrol 142
- Trigger 51/101 – Dimethylcarbamoyl Chloride 144
- Trigger 52/101 – 1,2-Dimethylhydrazine 146
- Trigger 53/101 – Dimethylvinyl Chloride 149
- Trigger 54/101 – N,N-Dimethyl-p-toluidine 152
- Trigger 55/101 – 1,4-Dioxane 155
- Trigger 56/101 – Epichlorohydrin 158
- Trigger 57/101 – Erionite 160
- Trigger 58/101 – Ethylbenzene 161
- Trigger 59/101 – Ethylene Oxide (EO) 163
- Trigger 60/101 – Etoposide 165
- Trigger 61/101 – Hexachloro-1,3-butadiene 167
- Trigger 62/101 – Indium Phosphide 168
- Trigger 63/101 – Isoprene 170
- Trigger 64/101 – Kaposi's Sarcoma Herpesvirus 172
- Trigger 65/101 – Leather Dust 174
- Trigger 66/101 – Melphalan 176
- Trigger 67/101 – 4,4'-Methylenebis(2-chloroaniline) 178
- Trigger 68/101 – 2,4,6-Trichlorophenol (TCP) 180
- Trigger 69/101 – Nitrogen Mustard 182
- Trigger 70/101 – Antimony Trioxide 183
- Trigger 71/101 – Arsenic 185
- Trigger 72/101 – Untreated Mineral Oils 187
- Trigger 73/101 – Nickel Compounds 190
- Trigger 74/101 – Amitrole 193
- Trigger 75/101 – Basic Red 9 Monohydrochloride 195
- Trigger 76/101 – Acetaldehyde 196
- Trigger 77/101 – 1-Bromopropane 198
- Trigger 78/101 – Chloramphenicol 199
- Trigger 79/101 – Dacarbazine 201
- Trigger 80/101 – Danthron 202
- Trigger 81/101 – Furan 204

Trigger 82/101 – Methylaziridine 207
Trigger 83/101 – Metronidazole 210
Trigger 84/101 – Nitrofen 212
Trigger 85/101 – Norethisterone 213
Trigger 86/101 – Oxymetholone 216
Trigger 87/101 – Reserpine 218
Trigger 88/101 – Selenium Sulfide 219
Trigger 89/101 – Vinyl Bromide 221
Trigger 90/101 – Tris(2,3-dibromopropyl) Phosphate 224
Trigger 91/101 – Toxaphene 226
Trigger 92/101 – Cyclophosphamide 228
Trigger 93/101 – Azathioprine 229
Trigger 94/101 – Malathion 230
Trigger 95/101 – Glyphosate 232
Trigger 96/101 – Glycidol 234
Trigger 97/101 – Ciclosporin 235
Trigger 98/101 – N-Nitrosodimethylamine 237
Trigger 99/101 – Benzene 238
Trigger 100/101 – Butylated hydroxyanisole (BHA) 241
Trigger 101/101 – Isobutyl Nitrite 243

CHAPTER 14: EXAMINING THE TRIGGERS 245
CHAPTER 15: FINAL THOUGHTS 248
REFERENCES 250

Unraveling the Origins: Exploring 101 Triggers of Cancer

INTRODUCTION

Growing up as the son of a science teacher, I've always had a passion for science. During my senior year of high school, I recall my science teacher discussing cancer. At that time, I imagined one day discovering a cure for cancer. However, I later learned a crucial truth: it's scientifically and mathematically impossible to cure an ailment while perpetuating its cause simultaneously. This creates a paradoxical situation. For instance, if smoking can lead to lung cancer and one continues to smoke, treating lung cancer without addressing smoking doesn't truly resolve the issue. The key to solving such problems lies in understanding its origins to avoid repeating initial mistakes. This concept echoes Sir Isaac Newton's famous principle: "For every action, there is an equal and opposite reaction," which underpins our understanding of how objects interact through Newton's Third Law of Motion.

Traditional medicine often times ignores root cause analysis which is ensuring that solutions address the fundamental causes of the problem rather than just the symptoms. This book focuses on exploring 101 triggers of cancer. "An ounce of prevention is worth a pound of cure" (Benjamin Franklin, 1735), which is a familiar maxim and a fundamental tenet of the field of prevention science.

In 1939 German scientist Franz H. Müller published a study showing a higher incidence of lung cancer among smokers. The year is now 2025, eighty-six years later and we are still faced with the same problem; lung cancer is still highly diagnosed. Simply put, man cannot compete with the laws of physics. Will there ever be a true 'cure' for cancer? Perhaps, but it will require addressing the root causes—those initial actions that are often overlooked in traditional medicine.

CHAPTER 1: WHAT IS CANCER?

Cancer is a multifaceted disease characterized by the abnormal and chaotic growth of cells within the body. This aberrant growth, known as neoplasia, results from genetic mutations that disrupt the normal regulatory mechanisms governing cell division and growth. These mutations can arise spontaneously or be triggered by various factors such as exposure to carcinogens, genetic predisposition, or viral infections.

Fundamentally, cancer manifests when cells acquire the ability to proliferate uncontrollably, forming masses or tumors. These tumors can be benign, remaining localized and non-invasive, or malignant, invading surrounding tissues and potentially spreading to other parts of the body through a process called metastasis. Cancer cells often exhibit altered metabolism, evasion of immune surveillance, and the ability to induce angiogenesis (the formation of new blood vessels) to sustain their growth.

The clinical manifestations of cancer vary widely depending on the type and location of the tumor, as well as its stage of progression. Symptoms may include unexplained weight loss, fatigue, pain, changes in bowel or bladder habits, persistent cough, and unusual bleeding or discharge. Diagnosis typically involves a combination of imaging studies (such as X-rays, CT scans, or MRIs), laboratory tests (including blood tests and tumor markers), and often biopsy to examine tissue under a microscope.

Free Radicals

A free radical is an atom, molecule (two or more atoms), or ion that has an unpaired electron in its outer shell, making it highly reactive and unstable. Because electrons prefer to be in pairs, free radicals seek to steal or donate an electron from or to other molecules to stabilize themselves. This process can cause a chain reaction of damage to cells, proteins, and DNA.

In the human body, free radicals are produced naturally as byproducts of normal metabolic processes, such as when the body uses oxygen to produce energy. However, they can also be introduced from external sources, like pollution, radiation, cigarette smoke, and certain **chemicals**.

While free radicals play a role in some necessary bodily functions, such as fighting infections, an excess of free radicals can lead to oxidative stress, which is linked to aging and various diseases, including cancer, heart disease, and neurodegenerative disorders. Antioxidants are substances that can neutralize free radicals by donating an electron, thereby preventing them from causing harm.

In summary, free radicals can initiate and promote the development of cancer by damaging DNA, disrupting normal cell regulation, and promoting a cellular environment that favors uncontrolled growth and division. Antioxidants, which neutralize free radicals, are one of the body's defenses against this process, helping to protect cells from oxidative stress and potentially reducing the risk of cancer.

Cancer Treatment

Treatment strategies for cancer are diverse and may include surgery to remove tumors and sometimes palliative care to alleviate symptoms and improve quality of life. The prognosis for cancer patients varies greatly depending on factors such as the type and stage of cancer, overall health, and response to treatment.

There are hundreds of drugs available to treat cancer, each designed to target different types of cancer and various stages of the disease. These drugs can be broadly categorized into several groups:

1. **Chemotherapy**: Traditional drugs that kill or inhibit the growth of rapidly dividing cancer cells.

2. **Radiation/Targeted Therapy**: Drugs that target specific molecules involved in cancer cell growth and survival.

3. **Immunotherapy**: Drugs that help the body's immune system recognize and fight cancer cells.

4. **Hormone Therapy**: Drugs that block or lower the amount of hormones in the body to slow or stop the growth of hormone-sensitive cancers.

5. **Monoclonal Antibodies**: Lab-made molecules that can bind to specific targets on cancer cells.

6. **Bone Marrow and Stem Cell Transplantation**: Procedures that restore blood-forming stem cells in patients who have had theirs destroyed by high doses of chemotherapy or radiation therapy

There are also hundreds of herbs and plants that have been studied for their potential to treat cancer or to alleviate the side effects of conventional cancer treatments. These studies range from basic laboratory research to clinical trials.

The number of herbs studied for cancer is large, and the research spans a broad spectrum of scientific rigor. While herbs have shown results in preclinical studies, translating these findings into effective and safe treatments for cancer in humans is said to be "complex" and requires extensive clinical trials. Additionally, the use of herbs in cancer treatment should always be discussed with healthcare professionals to avoid potential interactions with conventional treatments

Cancer Classification

Cancer is typically classified into stages to describe the extent of the disease in the body. These stages help determine the prognosis and the most appropriate treatment options. The most commonly used staging system is the TNM system, developed by the American Joint Committee on Cancer (AJCC). The stages are generally described as follows:

1. Stage 0 (Carcinoma in Situ)

Abnormal cells are present but have not spread to nearby tissue. This stage is considered pre-cancerous or early cancer. The cancer cells are still in the place where they started and have not spread.

2. Stage I (Early Stage)

Cancer is small and has only spread a little into nearby tissues. It has not spread to lymph nodes or other parts of the body. Often referred to as localized cancer, the tumor is generally small and can be surgically removed.

3. Stage II and III (Regional Spread)

Cancer is larger and has grown more deeply into nearby tissues. It may have spread to lymph nodes but not to other parts of the body.

- **Stage II**: Larger tumor size and/or spread to nearby lymph nodes.

- **Stage III**: Even larger tumors and/or extensive involvement of nearby lymph nodes.

4. Stage IV (Distant Spread)

Cancer has spread to other parts of the body (metastasis). This stage is also known as advanced or metastatic cancer. It indicates that the cancer has spread to distant organs or tissues.

Summary of the TNM System:

- **T (Tumor)**: Describes the size of the original tumor and whether it has invaded nearby tissue.
- **N (Node)**: Describes the extent of spread to nearby lymph nodes.
- **M (Metastasis)**: Describes whether the cancer has spread to other parts of the body.

Each of these components is assigned a number or letter to indicate the severity or extent of the disease. For example, T1N0M0 would indicate a small tumor with no lymph node involvement and no distant metastasis.

Understanding the stage of cancer is crucial for determining the most effective treatment plan and predicting the likely outcome for the patient.

CHAPTER 2: A BRIEF HISTORY OF CANCER

The history of cancer spans millennia, reflecting a gradual evolution in our understanding, perception, and treatment of this disease. Ancient medical texts from Egypt, dating back to around 3000 BC, contain descriptions of tumors that were likely cancerous. Throughout antiquity, cancer was often viewed fatalistically, associated with spiritual or supernatural causes, and treated with a combination of herbal remedies, surgery, and sometimes cautery (burning a part of the body).

Hippocrates (circa 460-370 BC) proposed that diseases, including cancer, arose from imbalances in bodily fluids, or humors. The term "cancer" comes from the Greek physician Hippocrates, who used the word "karkinos" (crab) to describe tumors because of their appearance. This theory persisted for centuries, influencing medical thought during the Roman Empire and the Middle Ages, where surgical interventions were occasionally attempted to remove tumors.

During the Renaissance period, there was a gradual shift towards more scientific inquiry and anatomical understanding. In the 17th century, William Harvey's discovery of the circulation of blood laid a foundation for understanding how diseases might spread within the body, including cancer. However, prevailing beliefs about disease causation remained largely rooted in humoral theory and metaphysical concepts.

Humoral theory, also known as the theory of the four humors, is an ancient medical concept that suggests that the human body is governed by four fluids or "humors": blood, phlegm, black bile, and yellow bile. This theory dominated Western medicine until the advent of modern medical science in the 19th century.

The 19th century marked a significant turning point with the advent of microscopy and the understanding that cells were the building blocks of all living organisms. In 1838, Johannes Müller proposed the theory that cancer arises from cells, a concept further developed by Rudolf Virchow, who emphasized the importance of pathological changes at the cellular level. This era also saw the first systematic classification of tumors based on their microscopic appearance.

The 20th century brought unprecedented advancements in cancer research and treatment. The discovery of X-rays by Wilhelm Roentgen in 1895 revolutionized diagnosis and enabled the visualization of tumors within the body. In the early 1900s, the identification of carcinogens such as tobacco smoke and occupational hazards led to a deeper understanding of environmental factors contributing to cancer development.

The mid-20th century witnessed breakthroughs in chemotherapy and radiation therapy, providing new tools to combat cancer. The development of antibiotics and improved surgical techniques also contributed to better outcomes for cancer patients. The discovery of DNA's structure by James Watson and Francis Crick in 1953 paved the way for understanding genetic mutations underlying cancer, leading to the field of molecular oncology and targeted therapies.

Today, cancer remains a formidable "challenge", with ongoing efforts focused on early detection, prevention strategies, and innovative treatments tailored to individual genetic profiles. The history of cancer underscores the enduring quest to unravel its complexities, offering hope for continued progress in reducing its burden on individuals and societies worldwide.

CHAPTER 3: WHAT IS A CARCINOGEN?

The term "carcinogen" comes from the Greek words "karkinos" (καρκίνος), meaning "crab" or "cancer," and "genes" (γενής), meaning "born of" or "producing." Genes (γενής) is a Greek suffix meaning "born of" or "producing." When combined, "carcinogen" literally means "producing cancer."

A carcinogen is any substance, radiation, or agent that is capable of causing cancer in living tissues or cells. Carcinogens can be found in various forms, including **chemicals**, physical agents, biological agents, and environmental factors. They can cause changes in the genetic material of cells (DNA) that lead to the development of cancer.

Carcinogens can be classified into several categories:

Chemical carcinogens: These are substances such as certain chemicals found in tobacco smoke (e.g., polycyclic aromatic hydrocarbons), industrial chemicals (e.g., benzene), pesticides, and certain food additives (e.g., nitrites) that have been shown to increase the risk of cancer.

Environmental carcinogens: These include pollutants in the air, water, and soil (e.g., asbestos fibers, arsenic, radon gas) that can be carcinogenic when exposed to humans over time.

Physical carcinogens: These are agents such as ionizing radiation (e.g., X-rays, gamma rays) and ultraviolet (UV) radiation from sunlight or tanning beds that can damage DNA and increase the risk of cancer.

Biological carcinogens: These are infectious agents such as certain viruses (e.g., human papillomavirus, hepatitis B and C viruses) and bacteria (e.g., Helicobacter pylori) that can cause chronic infections and inflammation, leading to cancer development.

It's important to note that not all exposure to carcinogens will result in cancer, and individual susceptibility can vary. Additionally, the level and duration of exposure, as well as other factors such as genetic predisposition and lifestyle choices, can influence the likelihood of cancer development. Avoiding or minimizing exposure to known carcinogens is an essential part of cancer prevention efforts.

The National Toxicology Program (NTP) is a part of the U.S. Department of Health and Human Services and is responsible for evaluating the potential health effects of exposure to various substances, including carcinogens. One of the key reports published by the NTP is the "Report on Carcinogens" (RoC). There are 15 editions of the Report on Carcinogens (RoC). The 15th Report, includes 256 substances that are known or reasonably anticipated to cause cancer in humans.

The Report on Carcinogens is a congressionally mandated, science-based document that identifies substances known to be human carcinogens or reasonably anticipated to be human carcinogens based on scientific evidence. The report is intended to provide health professionals, policymakers, and the **public** with information about substances that may pose a cancer risk.

What one will notice that is **not** listed as a carcinogen, but we often times hear people say are the following:

1. Genetics (It runs in my family)
2. Bad Luck
3. I'm being tested.

Unraveling the Origins: Exploring 101 Triggers of Cancer

It is important to understand the correlation of cause and effect. Genetics is not a verb/action; it is a noun. "Genetics" is a term for a scientific field of study and cannot function as a verb.

Simply put, nouns don't cause cancer. Dr. Dean Omish, who wrote the book The Spectrum, chronicled a UCLA study utilized food to alter genetic markers for prostate cancer. He concluded that "although you can't change your genes you can alter how they are expressed." There is an entire scientific field based on gene expressions. Epigenetics is the study of changes in gene expression or cellular phenotype that do not involve alterations in the DNA sequence. These changes can be influenced by various environmental factors, lifestyle choices, and developmental stages, and they can affect how genes are turned on or off. Factors such as diet, stress, **toxins**, and physical activity can lead to epigenetic changes. Exposure to certain **chemicals** can result in DNA methylation patterns that increase the risk of cancer.

The concept of "luck" as understood in contemporary terms—an unpredictable and often beneficial force affecting events—doesn't have a direct equivalent in any holy scriptures or religious books. God nor the Devil is creating cancer inside of our body. We have free will and parish due to lack of knowledge. All 101 factors in this book are derived from actions — cause and effect. The contents in this book are not my opinions; I'm simply a messenger.

CHAPTER 4. THE COST OF CANCER

The cost of cancer in the United States is substantial, encompassing direct medical costs, indirect costs due to loss of productivity, and intangible costs related to pain and suffering. The National Cancer Institute (NCI) estimated that the direct medical costs for cancer care in the U.S. were approximately $208.9 billion in 2020. Indirect costs are associated with lost productivity due to illness and premature death. A study published in the Journal of the National Cancer Institute in 2020 estimated that the annual cost of productivity losses due to cancer-related mortality was approximately $94.4 billion. When combining direct medical costs and indirect costs, the total economic burden of cancer in the U.S. was estimated to be over $300 billion annually as of recent years. The cost of cancer care is expected to increase in the coming years due to an aging population, advances in cancer treatments, and rising healthcare costs. A study published in the Journal of the National Cancer Institute in 2011 projected that the cost of cancer care could reach $246 billion by 2030.

According to a report by the American Cancer Society and the World Economic Forum in 2010, the total global economic cost of cancer was estimated at approximately $1.16 trillion per year. A study published in the Lancet in 2016 estimated that the productivity losses due to cancer mortality alone were around $116 billion annually. A study by the World Health Organization (WHO) projected that by 2030, the global cancer burden could reach $458 billion in annual direct medical costs alone.

Unraveling the Origins: Exploring 101 Triggers of Cancer

These figures illustrate the significant financial impact of cancer on the U.S. healthcare system and economy. The costs highlight the importance of effective cancer prevention, early detection, and efficient treatment strategies to manage and potentially reduce this economic burden.

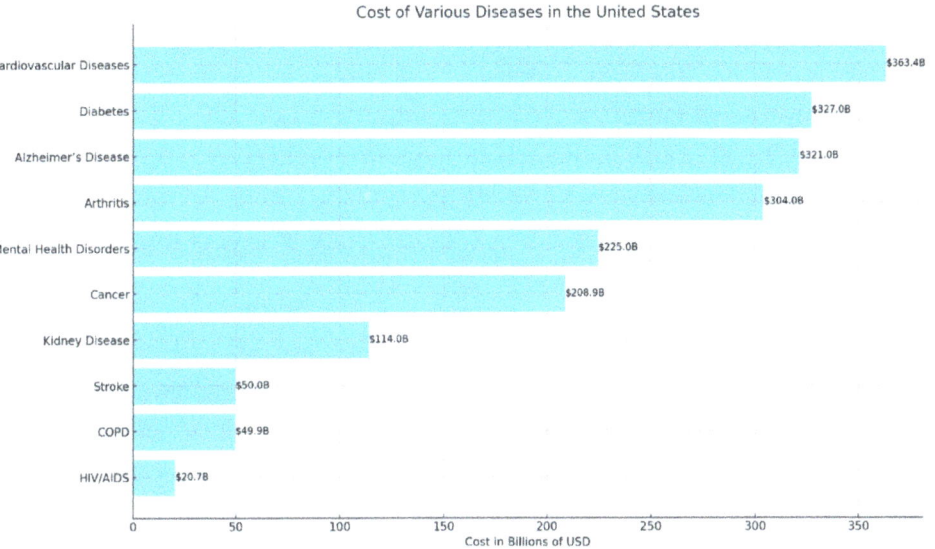

The cost of cancer treatment varies widely based on several factors. Initial treatment costs can range significantly: surgery typically costs between $15,000 and $40,000, radiation therapy between $10,000 and $50,000, chemotherapy from $10,000 to $200,000 per year depending on the drugs and frequency of treatment, and immunotherapy from $150,000 to $200,000 per year. Ongoing treatment costs, including follow-up visits, additional tests, and ongoing medication, can add thousands of dollars annually. Even with insurance, patients may face significant out-of-pocket costs, including copayments, coinsurance, and deductibles, which can range from a few thousand to tens of thousands of dollars.

CHAPTER 5: CANCER STATISTICS

According to estimates from the American Cancer Society (ACS) based on data from the United States, approximately 39.5% of men and women will be diagnosed with cancer at some point during their lifetime. This statistic means that nearly 2 in 5 people will develop cancer at some stage in their lives. Overall, cancer rates have been increasing globally over the past few decades, primarily due to factors such as population growth, aging populations, changes in lifestyle and environmental exposures. However, it's essential to consider the specific trends for different types of cancer and populations when examining cancer incidence rates.

Listing all the types of cancer would be an exhaustive task given the vast number of subtypes and variations. However, some of the most common types of cancer, categorized by the organ or tissue where they originate:

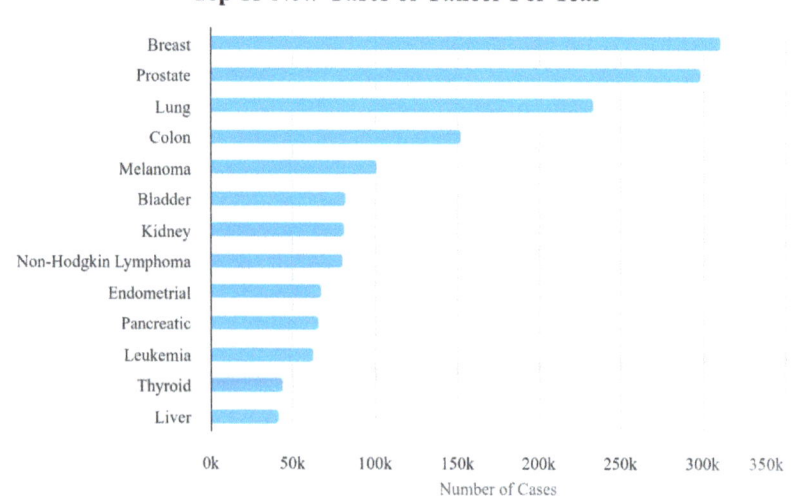

Unraveling the Origins: Exploring 101 Triggers of Cancer

This list is not exhaustive, and there are many other types of cancer that can affect different parts of the body. Each type of cancer can have multiple subtypes and variations, making the classification complex. This list of common cancer types includes cancers that are diagnosed with the greatest frequency in the United States

1. Breast cancer (311,000 per year)
2. Prostate cancer (299,000 per year)
3. Lung cancer (235,000 per year)
4. Colon and Rectal cancer (152,000 per year)
5. Skin cancer (101,00 per year)
6. Bladder cancer (83,000 per year)
7. Kidney cancer (82,000 per year)
8. Lymphoma (81,000 per year)
9. Endometrial cancer (68,000 per year)
10. Pancreatic cancer (66,000 per year)
11. Leukemia cancer (63,000 per year)
12. Thyroid cancer (44,000 per year)
13. Liver cancer (42,000 per year)

CHAPTER 6: CANCER RESEARCH REPORTS

The Report on Carcinogens (RoC) is a public health document prepared by the National Toxicology Program (NTP) in the United States. It identifies substances, both chemical and biological, that are known or reasonably anticipated to cause cancer in humans. The RoC is published biennially and serves as a critical resource for researchers, policymakers, and the **public** to understand and address potential cancer risks associated with various substances. It categorizes substances based on scientific evidence from studies on humans and animals regarding their carcinogenicity. The Report on Carcinogens (RoC) was established in 1980 by the United States Congress as a requirement of the Public Health Service Act.

The RoC categorizes carcinogenic substances into two main groups:

1. Known Human Carcinogens: These are substances for which there is sufficient evidence from human studies or, in some cases, strong evidence from animal studies to conclude that they can cause cancer in humans.

2. Reasonably Anticipated Human Carcinogens: These are substances for which there is limited evidence from human studies or sufficient evidence from animal studies to suggest they may increase the risk of cancer in humans.

The NTP periodically updates the Report on Carcinogens to reflect new scientific findings and advancements in cancer research. The first edition was released in 1980 and contained 26 known carcinogens. The 15th edition, which is the latest edition of the Report on Carcinogens provides information on over 250

Unraveling the Origins: Exploring 101 Triggers of Cancer

substances, including chemicals, biological agents, and other environmental factors.

It's important to note that the inclusion of a substance in the Report on Carcinogens does not necessarily mean that exposure to that substance will cause cancer in every individual or under all circumstances. The report is intended to inform risk assessment and management efforts to reduce exposures to substances that may pose a cancer risk. Most of the triggers written in this book is derived from The Report on Carcinogens.

There are also other references and publications including the Environmental Protection Agency (EPA), Agency for Toxic Substances and Disease Registry (ATSDR), World Heal Organization (WHO), European Chemicals Agency (ECHA), Occupational Safety and Health Administration (OSHA), National Cancer Institute (NCI), and the European Food Safety Authority (EFSA). These documents and reports are similar to the "Report on Carcinogens" in that they provide scientific evaluations and assessments of substances and exposures that may cause cancer, thereby informing public health policies, regulatory actions, and research priorities.

There isn't a precise number of known toxic chemicals, as new substances are continually being discovered and their toxicological properties assessed. However, there are thousands of **chemicals** known to be toxic to humans and other organisms. These include heavy metals like lead and mercury, pesticides, industrial chemicals, and various pollutants. Many of these substances can have harmful effects on health and the environment at certain concentrations or under specific exposure conditions.

CHAPTER 7: ANIMAL TESTING

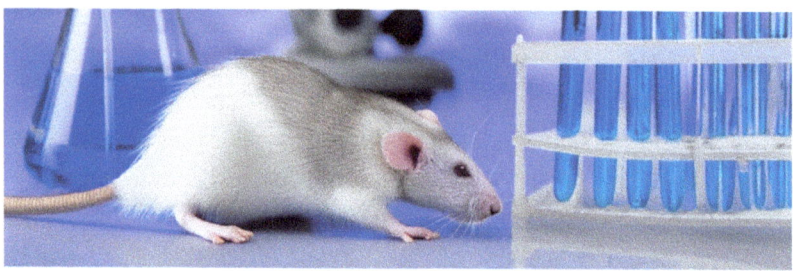

Estimating the exact number of animals used in laboratory testing worldwide and the number that die each year can be challenging due to variations in reporting standards, regulatory requirements, and research practices across different countries and institutions. However, estimates from various sources provide some insights:

1. **United States**: According to the U.S. Department of Agriculture (USDA), over 1 million animals are used annually for research purposes, including testing. The exact number that dies from testing each year is not specified separately but is included in the overall count of animals used.

2. **European Union**: In the EU, statistics are collected and reported annually under the Directive 2010/63/EU, which regulates the use of animals in scientific research. In 2017, approximately 9.39 million animals were used across the EU member states for research purposes, including testing.

3. **Global Estimates**: Globally, estimates suggest that tens of millions of animals are used each year in research, testing, and education. This includes a wide range of animals from rodents (mice and rats) to larger mammals (like dogs, cats, and primates).

Unraveling the Origins: Exploring 101 Triggers of Cancer

Testing for toxicity using animals typically involves several steps, which can vary depending on the specific substance being tested and regulatory requirements. Here's a general outline of the process:

1. **Test Selection**: Researchers select appropriate animal species for testing based on factors such as the type of substance, intended use, and regulatory guidelines. Common animals used include mice, rats, rabbits, and sometimes larger animals like dogs or primates.

2. **Dose Selection**: Researchers determine appropriate doses of the substance to administer to the animals. This often includes selecting a range of doses to observe potential effects across different exposure levels.

3. **Administration**: The substance is administered to the animals, usually through ingestion, inhalation, or injection, depending on the substance's intended route of exposure (e.g., oral, dermal).

4. **Observation Period**: Animals are observed over a specified period, which can range from hours to weeks or months, depending on the expected timeframe for toxicity effects to manifest.

5. **Monitoring**: Throughout the observation period, researchers closely monitor the animals for signs of toxicity, including behavioral changes, physiological effects, and any adverse health outcomes.

6. **Data Collection**: Detailed records are kept of all observations, including the onset and severity of any symptoms, changes in body weight, and results of pathological examinations if the

animals are sacrificed for tissue analysis.

7. **Analysis**: Data collected from the study are analyzed to determine the substance's toxicity profile, including the LD50 (median lethal dose) if applicable, and other measures of toxicity such as NOAEL (no observed adverse effect level) or LOAEL (lowest observed adverse effect level).

8. **Regulatory Submission**: If required, study results are submitted to regulatory agencies for review as part of the approval process for substances intended for human or animal use.

9. **Ethical Considerations**: Throughout the process, ethical considerations regarding the use of animals in testing are paramount, with efforts made to minimize suffering and use alternatives when possible.

It's important to note that there is ongoing debate and efforts within the scientific community to reduce the use of animals in toxicity testing through alternative methods such as in vitro tests and computer modeling.

CHAPTER 8: CHEMICALS AND TOXICITY

As you read this book, you will notice that most carcinogens are classified as **chemical** carcinogens. Chemicals, especially **synthetic** ones, can be a hazard to human health because they don't interact well with our natural biological systems. These chemicals interfere with cellular processes that regulate cell growth and division.

"Synthetic" refers to something that is made by chemical or biological processes, rather than being naturally occurring. In other words, synthetic substances are produced artificially in a laboratory or manufacturing facility, often through chemical reactions or biological processes, rather than being derived directly from natural sources.

In the context of organic chemistry, synthetic compounds are often created through the synthesis of organic molecules from simpler starting materials using chemical reactions. This process allows chemists to design and create new compounds with desired properties for various applications, including pharmaceuticals, agrochemicals, materials science, and more.

The majority of pharmaceutical drugs, and all substances that are man-made are synthesized from organic compounds, which can be derived from natural sources like plants, animals, fungi, or bacteria. These compounds serve as the active ingredients in medications, and they undergo various processes such as extraction, purification, and **chemical modification** to create pharmaceutical formulations. As a certified nutritionist, herbalist and health and wellness coach, I know that most pharmaceutical drugs are synthetic versions of nature. You will notice that many chemotherapy drugs are themselves a known carcinogen because their chemical structure is foreign to the body and the compounds are toxic. This book does not focus much on alternative solutions to heal cancer naturally due to the fact that knowing what causes cancer is the first half of the battle. Our first objective is to understand the root cause of cancer; later we can focus on reversing these effects.

Toxins can interact with DNA in several ways, potentially leading to mutations, cancer, and other health issues. Some toxins directly bind to DNA and form DNA adducts, which are covalent bonds between the toxin and DNA bases. Examples include aflatoxins, found in contaminated food, and benzo[a]pyrene, found in tobacco smoke. Other toxins generate reactive oxygen species (ROS) that cause oxidative damage to DNA, resulting in base modifications, strand breaks, and crosslinking. Heavy metals like arsenic and cadmium, and chemicals like hydrogen peroxide, are examples of such toxins.

Certain toxins intercalate between DNA base pairs, disrupting the DNA structure and interfering with replication and transcription. Additionally, toxins can include base analogs, which are structurally similar to DNA bases and get incorporated into DNA during replication, leading to mutations. Toxins can also cause single-strand or double-strand breaks in DNA, which can lead to cell death if not properly repaired.

Cells have mechanisms to detect and repair DNA damage caused by toxins, including DNA repair pathways like base excision repair (BER), nucleotide excision repair (NER), mismatch repair (MMR), and homologous recombination (HR). Cells can also halt the cell cycle to repair damage before proceeding or undergo programmed cell death (apoptosis) if the damage is irreparable. The impact of toxin interaction with DNA can vary based on the type of toxin, exposure level, and the efficiency of the cellular repair mechanisms.

Unraveling the Origins: Exploring 101 Triggers of Cancer

CHAPTER 9: MY TOXICITY REPORT

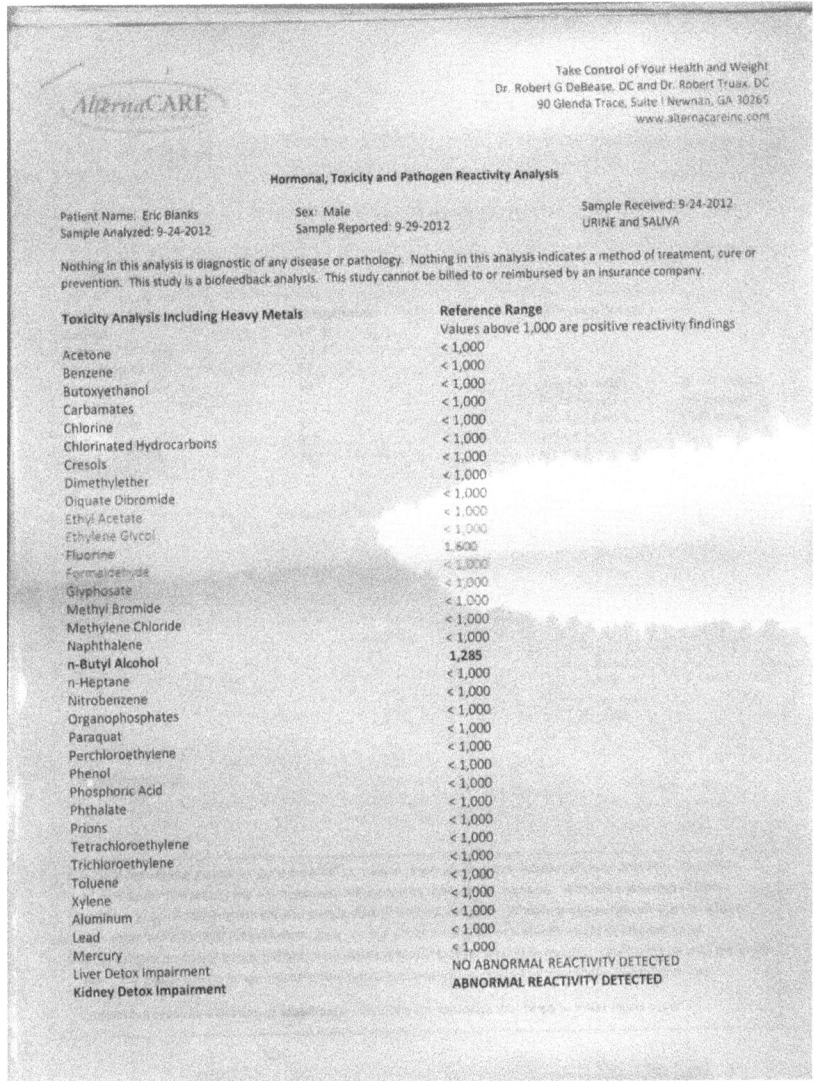

In 2006, I was diagnosed with Graves' Disease, which is considered an "incurable disease." Graves' disease is an autoimmune disorder that affects the thyroid gland, causing it to produce too much thyroid hormone (hyperthyroidism). It is the most common cause of hyperthyroidism and is named after Robert Graves, an Irish doctor who first described the condition in the early 19th century. I was told by my Endocrinologist that I would probably be on medication for my entire life. Shortly after being diagnosed, I opted into retrieving radioactive iodine therapy. Radioactive iodine is taken orally and absorbed by the thyroid gland, where it destroys thyroid cells. I was then placed on a synthetic thyroid hormone medication which is called levothyroxine. Levothyroxine is a synthetic form of the thyroid hormone thyroxine (T4), which is naturally produced by the thyroid gland. It is commonly used as a replacement therapy in individuals with hypothyroidism (underactive thyroid), a condition where the thyroid gland does not produce enough thyroid hormone.

After being introduced to holistic medicine, I discovered the possibility of re-growing my thyroid, potentially eliminating the need for synthetic hormones. When I shared my plans with my endocrinologist, he chuckled and stated, "Homeopathic medicine doesn't work." His skepticism motivated me to explore further. Through my research, I found a holistic healthcare facility and began my journey of self-healing. One of the first steps they took was ordering a toxicity report, which is shown on the previous page.

If you examine the report, you will notice that my toxicity lab shows that I have high levels of fluorine and n-Butyl Alcohol. n-Butyl alcohol, also known as 1-butanol or butan-1-ol is used in manufacturing varnishes, paints, coatings, and resins. It also serves as a building block in the synthesis of various pharmaceutical compounds and used as a fuel or blended with gasoline to improve combustion and reduce emissions. Technically n-Butyl Alcohol is not listed as a known carcinogen based on the Report on Carcinogens. However, under EPA's Guidelines for Carcinogen Risk Assessment (U.S. EPA, 2005), tert-butyl alcohol has "suggestive evidence of carcinogenic potential" for all routes of exposure based on some evidence in animals.

n-Butyl Alcohol is related to tert-Butyl alcohol. Tert-Butyl alcohol is the simplest tertiary alcohol. Its isomers are 1-butanol, isobutanol, and butan-2-ol. Both are forms of butanol. Exposure to tert-butanol occurs primarily through breathing air containing tert-butanol vapors and consuming contaminated water or foods. Exposure can also occur through direct skin contact. Evidence is suggestive of carcinogenic potential for tert-butanol, based on thyroid tumors in male and female mice and renal tumors in male rats. A quantitative estimate of carcinogenic potential from oral exposure to tert-butanol was based on the increased incidence of thyroid follicular cell adenomas in female B6C3F1 mice and thyroid follicular cell adenomas and carcinomas in male B6C3F1 mice (NTP, 1995).

I also tested for higher-than-normal levels of Fluoride. Fluoride is commonly found in drinking water, dental products, and certain foods. It is known for its benefits in preventing dental cavities. Fluoride exposure in areas with low iodine levels may exacerbate iodine deficiency, leading to thyroid dysfunction. Fluoride can compete with iodine uptake by the thyroid gland, potentially reducing the production of thyroid hormones.

Fluoride has been shown to inhibit the activity of deiodinase enzymes, which are responsible for the conversion of the inactive thyroid hormone (T4) to the active form (T3). This can affect thyroid hormone levels and function. Animal studies have shown that high levels of fluoride can lead to thyroid dysfunction, including reduced thyroid hormone levels and goiter (enlarged thyroid gland).

World Health Organization (WHO) states that fluoride levels in drinking water up to 1.5 mg/L are safe and beneficial for dental health. They also acknowledge that excessive fluoride intake can cause health problems, including potential effects on the thyroid. The National Research Council (NRC) Report (2006) reviewed the evidence and concluded that fluoride exposure at high levels (above 4 mg/L) has the potential to impact thyroid function, particularly in individuals with iodine deficiency.

My toxicity report reveals the presence of two toxins that directly impacted my thyroid, with one identified as a potential carcinogen. These issues were not addressed or communicated to me by my endocrinologist. I am now off all thyroid medication, and my thyroid has regrown and is functioning normally. My body was able to self-heal once my root issues were addressed. Due to the focus of this book, my journey to a full thyroid recovery will be discussed separately.

My toxicity report was provided by Alternacare Weight Loss & Holistic Healthcare (www.alternacareinc.com), located in Newnan, GA. I am deeply grateful to Dr. Robert Debease, Dr. Robert Truax and Alternacare's entire staff for their support in overcoming my thyroid issues.

CHAPTER 10: WE KNOW THE CAUSE — YET WE DO LITTLE FOR PREVENTION

There are over 1,600 chemicals that are banned from cosmetics in the European Union while the FDA (Food and Drug Administration) has only banned a handful. The FDA is ~50% funded through user fees.

For example:

- **Prescription Drug User Fee Act (PDUFA):** Fees paid by pharmaceutical companies when they submit applications for new drugs or biologics.

- **Medical Device User Fee Amendments (MDUFA):** Fees paid by medical device companies for the review of device applications.

- **Generic Drug User Fee Amendments (GDUFA):** Fees paid by manufacturers of generic drugs for review of abbreviated new drug applications (ANDAs).

These user fees help supplement the FDA's budget and support faster review timelines for product approvals.

The relationship between lobbyists and the FDA can be complex and controversial, often involving efforts by various interest groups to influence FDA policies, regulations, and decisions. Here are some key aspects of this relationship:

1. **Advocacy and Influence:** Lobbyists represent different stakeholders, such as pharmaceutical companies, medical device manufacturers, consumer advocacy groups, and healthcare providers. They advocate for their clients' interests by providing information, analysis, and recommendations to

FDA officials and policymakers.

2. **Policy Development:** Lobbyists may participate in the FDA's rulemaking process by submitting comments on proposed regulations, attending public meetings, and engaging in discussions with FDA staff. They seek to shape policies that affect their industries or causes.

3. **Access to Information:** Lobbyists often have access to FDA officials and policymakers, which can provide them with insights into upcoming regulations, guidance documents, or other decisions. This access allows them to better strategize their advocacy efforts.

4. **Financial Contributions:** Lobbyists and their clients may contribute to political campaigns of elected officials who oversee FDA activities or influence legislation that impacts the FDA's authority and funding.

The fees and influence make it very difficult for laws to be written and passed. Political scientists Martin Gilens of Princeton University and Benjamin I. Page of Northwestern University in their 2014 paper titled "Testing Theories of American Politics: Elites, Interest Groups, and Average Citizens" suggests that U.S. policy making is heavily influenced by economic elites and organized interest groups (like lobbyists), rather than the average citizen.

The study analyzed data from approximately 1,800 policy issues to determine whose preferences were most closely aligned with actual policy outcomes.

Unraveling the Origins: Exploring 101 Triggers of Cancer

The findings indicated that:

- Economic elites and organized business groups have substantial independent impacts on U.S. government policy.

- Average citizens and mass-based interest groups have little or no independent influence on policy outcomes.

This led to the conclusion that the U.S. operates more as an oligarchy than a democracy, with policy decisions often reflecting the preferences of the wealthy and well-connected rather than the broader public.

Politics is not the only ones to blame. People often participate in activities that are known to cause cancer. Substances like tobacco and alcohol can be highly addictive, making it difficult for individuals to quit despite knowing the risks. Also, smoking and drinking can be social activities that people engage in to fit in or bond with others. Eating certain foods provide immediate pleasure and enjoyment. The long-term risks can seem abstract compared to the immediate gratification. People often believe that the negative consequences of their actions won't happen to them. This optimism bias can lead to risky behaviors despite knowing the potential dangers.

CHAPTER 11: A TALE OF TWO CONSPIRACIES

Big Tobacco

Lung cancer was once extremely rare, to the point where doctors considered it a noteworthy anomaly. However, the mechanization and mass marketing of cigarettes in the late 19th century led to a global epidemic of lung cancer. By the 1940s and 1950s, cigarettes were identified as the primary cause of this epidemic through a combination of epidemiological studies, animal experiments, cellular pathology, and chemical analysis. In 1954, Philip Morris Vice President George Weissman stated that if the company had any suspicion or knowledge that their product was harmful to consumers, they would **_cease operations immediately_**. However, senior scientists and executives at tobacco companies were aware of the potential cancer risk associated with smoking as early as the 1940s, and by the late 1950s, most had accepted that smoking caused cancer. For most of the past 100 years, cigarette manufacturers have told smokers that their products were not proven to be injurious to health.

Despite this evidence, cigarette manufacturers launched a coordinated effort to refute these findings in order to protect their sales. Their propaganda efforts were effective, as evidenced by internal tobacco industry documents showing the impact of their denialist campaigns. Even as late as 1960, only one-third of U.S. doctors were convinced that cigarettes were harmful. Cigarettes remain the deadliest product in human history.

In 1994, the leaders of major U.S. tobacco companies testified before Congress, claiming that the evidence linking cigarette smoking to diseases like cancer and heart disease was inconclusive, that cigarettes were not addictive, and that they did not market to children. However, less than a month after this testimony, a box containing confidential documents from the Brown & Williamson Tobacco Corporation was delivered to the University of California at San Francisco. These documents revealed that the tobacco industry had known for decades that cigarettes caused premature death, recognized their addictive nature, and that their scientific research programs on smoking and health were fraudulent.

In 1955, Dr. Clarence Little, the first Scientific Director of TIRC, appeared on the Edward R. Murrow show and was asked, "Dr. Little have any cancer-causing agents been identified in cigarettes?" Dr. Little replied, "No. None whatever, either in cigarettes or in any product of smoking, as such." Dr. Little was also asked, "Suppose the tremendous amount of research going on were to reveal that there is a cancer causing agent in cigarettes, what then?" Dr. Little replied, "It would be made public immediately and just as broadly as we could make it, and then efforts would be taken to attempt to remove that substance or substances"

Big Pharma

With a diverse portfolio including pharmaceuticals, medical devices, and consumer health products, Johnson & Johnson is a major player in the global healthcare market. As of mid-2024, Johnson & Johnson's market capitalization is approximately $450 billion. Johnson & Johnson has acquired numerous companies over its long history and has a substantial number of subsidiaries. As of 2024, J&J has over 250 operating companies in more than 60 countries.

Johnson & Johnson knew since the late 1950s that the talc used in its iconic baby powder was sometimes contaminated with asbestos, a substance known to cause ovarian cancer and mesothelioma. Despite this knowledge, J&J kept the contamination a secret from the public and regulators for decades. In 1976, while the U.S. Food and Drug Administration (FDA) was considering limits on asbestos in cosmetic talc products, J&J assured the agency that no asbestos was "detected in any sample" of talc produced between December 1972 and October 1973. They failed to disclose that at least three tests by different labs between 1972 and 1975 had found asbestos in their talc—one at rather high levels. Most of J&J's internal asbestos tests involved sampling only 1 pound of talc per 20 tons, as indicated in documents submitted to the FDA in 1971.

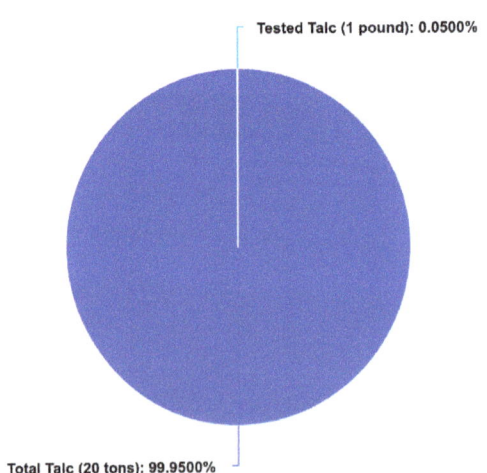

The pie chart shows the proportions between "Total Weight" (40000 pounds) and "Total Tested" (1 pound). The chart visually demonstrates the significant difference in size between the two items, with "Total Weight" occupying nearly the entire chart. The "Total Tested" represents approximately 0.0025%.

Unraveling the Origins: Exploring 101 Triggers of Cancer

In April 2020, a media exposé revealed that J&J increased marketing to African Americans and overweight women, aware of the asbestos-related health risks linked to their baby powder, as U.S. sales declined. A specific J&J memo suggested exploring ethnic (African American/Hispanic) market opportunities to grow the franchise. In October 2021, J&J filed for bankruptcy and created a subsidiary to handle the liabilities from the 40,000 lawsuits filed against them. Court documents revealed J&J's 1970s talc testing predominantly involved Black inmates. Previously unsealed trial documents showed the company funded experiments primarily on Black men, comparing the effects of talc and asbestos on their skin. In one study, inmates were injected with potentially cancer-causing asbestos to compare its effects on their skin to those of talc.

On August 11, 2022, Johnson & Johnson announced they would cease global sales of talc-based baby powder and transition to a safer corn-starch-based formula for all customers by 2023.

CHAPTER 12: LAWS AND CANCER WARNINGS

The history of cancer warnings is intertwined with the evolving understanding of cancer's causes and the development of public health policies. The U.S. Surgeon General's report on smoking and health conclusively linked smoking with lung cancer and other diseases, leading to the first public health warnings on cigarette packages in 1966. Despite advancements, ensuring that the public understands, and heeds cancer warnings remains a challenge, particularly in combating misinformation and promoting preventive behaviors.

Below are warning laws and notices from different organizations from around the world.

United States:

Proposition 65 (California):

California's Proposition 65, also known as the Safe Drinking Water and Toxic Enforcement Act of 1986, is a landmark piece of legislation aimed at protecting California residents and the state's drinking water sources from chemicals known to cause cancer, birth defects, or other reproductive harm. Here's a brief history of Proposition 65:

1. **Enactment:** Proposition 65 was approved by California voters as a ballot initiative in November 1986. It was introduced in response to growing concerns about exposure to toxic chemicals in the environment, consumer products, and drinking water.

2. **Purpose:** The primary goals of Proposition 65 are to:

Unraveling the Origins: Exploring 101 Triggers of Cancer

- Inform consumers about potential exposures to chemicals known to cause cancer, birth defects, or other reproductive harm.
- Encourage businesses to reduce or eliminate the use of these chemicals in consumer products and workplaces.

3. **List of Chemicals:** Proposition 65 requires the State of California to maintain and update a list of chemicals known to cause cancer, birth defects, or other reproductive harm. As of 2024, the list includes over 900 chemicals.

4. **Warning Requirements:** Businesses with 10 or more employees that expose Californians to listed chemicals must provide clear and reasonable warnings before knowingly exposing individuals to these chemicals. Warnings can be provided on product labels, signage at workplaces, or notices distributed to affected populations.

5. **Litigation and Compliance:** Proposition 65 has led to numerous lawsuits filed by private individuals, advocacy groups, and the California Attorney General's office against businesses alleged to be in violation of its requirements. Settlements often include financial penalties and agreements to reformulate products to reduce chemical exposures.

6. **Impact and Controversy:** While Proposition 65 has been credited with raising awareness about chemical exposures and prompting reformulations of consumer products, it has also faced criticism for potentially excessive litigation, compliance costs for businesses, and challenges in interpreting scientific evidence related to chemical risks.

Overall, Proposition 65 remains a significant environmental and consumer protection law in California, influencing product formulations, consumer purchasing decisions, and regulatory approaches to chemical safety nationwide.

OSHA Hazard Communication Standard (HCS):

European Union:

1. *CLP Regulation (Classification, Labelling, and Packaging):*

2. *REACH Regulation (Registration, Evaluation, Authorisation, and Restriction of Chemicals):*

Canada:

WHMIS (Workplace Hazardous Materials Information System):

Australia:

Work Health and Safety (WHS) Regulations:

International:

Globally Harmonized System (GHS):

These laws are designed to protect public health by ensuring that individuals are informed about potential cancer risks and can take appropriate precautions.

Unraveling the Origins: Exploring 101 Triggers of Cancer

CHAPTER 13: CANCER TRIGGERS

I have compiled a list of 101 carcinogens that have the potential to affect us today. There are well over 500 known carcinogens. Some are outlawed and no longer in circulation, yet they continue to pose risks due to their lingering effects in the environment. Additionally, many carcinogens are variants of other chemical compounds, so they were omitted from the list of triggers.

Over the past five years, I have researched each carcinogen closely. Without further ado, here is a list of substances that could potentially increase the risk of being diagnosed with cancer.

Trigger 1/101 – Tobacco Smoke

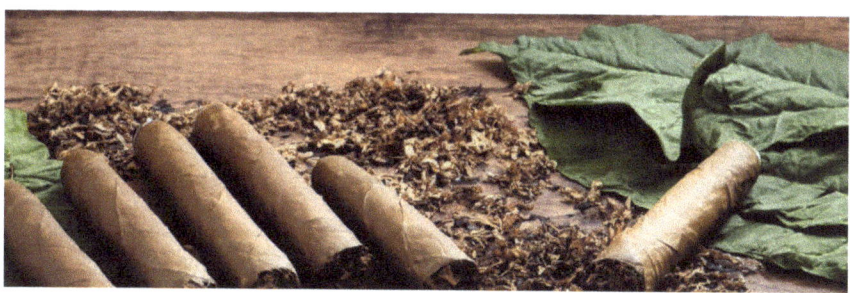

Report: 1st Report on Carcinogens
Carcinogen Category: chemical
Cancer Type(s): lung, throat, mouth, bladder, etc

Tobacco smoke is considered a carcinogen because it contains thousands of chemicals, many of which are known to be harmful to human health. Among these chemicals, at least 70 are known carcinogens, meaning they have been proven to cause cancer in humans or animals. Some of the key carcinogens found in tobacco smoke include:

1. **Nicotine**: While not a carcinogen itself, nicotine is addictive and keeps people smoking, exposing them to other harmful chemicals in tobacco smoke.

2. **Tar**: Tar is a sticky substance that forms when tobacco is burned. It contains numerous carcinogens, including polycyclic aromatic hydrocarbons (PAHs) and benzene.

3. **Polycyclic aromatic hydrocarbons (PAHs)**: PAHs are formed when organic material, such as tobacco, is burned. They are known to cause cancer in humans.

4. **Nitrosamines**: Nitrosamines are formed from nicotine and other tobacco components during the curing, processing, and smoking of tobacco. They are potent carcinogens.

5. **Formaldehyde**: Formaldehyde is a chemical used to preserve dead bodies. It is also found in tobacco smoke and is a known carcinogen.

6. **Acrolein**: Acrolein is a highly toxic and reactive substance found in tobacco smoke. It can damage DNA and is considered a carcinogen.

These chemicals are inhaled into the lungs when tobacco is smoked. They can cause damage to the DNA in cells, leading to the uncontrolled growth of cells characteristic of cancer. This damage can occur in various tissues throughout the body, explaining why smoking is associated with a wide range of cancers, including lung cancer, throat cancer, mouth cancer, bladder cancer, and others. Additionally, tobacco smoke not only affects smokers but also poses health risks to those exposed to secondhand smoke.

Unraveling the Origins: Exploring 101 Triggers of Cancer

Cigars typically contain tobacco. They are made from dried and fermented tobacco leaves, which are rolled tightly to form a cylindrical shape. Unlike cigarettes, which often contain shredded tobacco wrapped in paper, cigars are composed entirely of tobacco leaves.

It's important to note that like cigarettes, cigars also pose health risks due to the presence of tobacco and the chemicals produced when tobacco is burned. Cigar smoke contains many of the same harmful substances found in cigarette smoke, and cigar smoking is associated with health problems such as cancer, heart disease, and respiratory issues.

Hookah (also known as shisha, narghile, or waterpipe) usually contains tobacco. The tobacco used in hookahs is often flavored and mixed with molasses, honey, or fruit, creating a moist mixture that produces a lot of smoke when heated. The smoke passes through water before being inhaled, but it still contains nicotine, tar, and other harmful chemicals. Some hookah mixtures may be tobacco-free, using herbal substitutes instead, but these can still produce harmful smoke when burned. Hookah has gained significant popularity in recent years, particularly among young adults and in social settings.

Trigger 2/101 – Formaldehyde

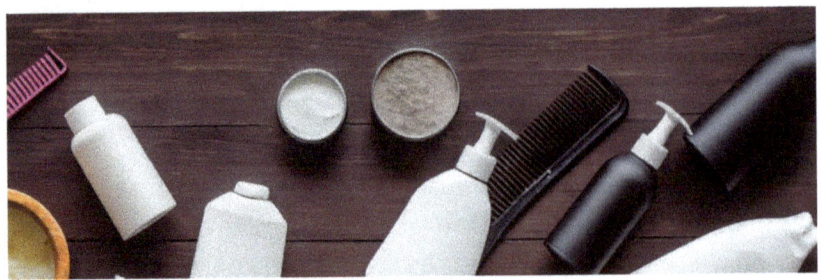

Report: 2nd Report on Carcinogens
Carcinogen Category: environment
Cancer Type(s): leukemia, sinonasal/nasal, head/neck/brain

Formaldehyde is a simple chemical compound made of hydrogen, oxygen, and carbon. It is naturally occurring and also widely used in industrial applications. Formaldehyde and formaldehyde-releasing agents are used in certain cosmetics and personal care products as preservatives to prevent microbial growth and extend shelf life. While the use of formaldehyde in cosmetics has declined in recent years due to safety concerns, it may still be found in some products.

Products may include:

1. **Nail Polish**: Formaldehyde and formaldehyde-releasing agents have historically been used in nail polish formulations to help prevent the growth of bacteria and fungi. However, many manufacturers have reformulated their nail polishes to be formaldehyde-free.

2. **Nail Hardeners**: Some nail hardeners may contain formaldehyde or formaldehyde-releasing agents to strengthen and protect the nails.

Unraveling the Origins: Exploring 101 Triggers of Cancer

3. **Hair Straightening Products**: Certain hair straightening treatments, such as Brazilian keratin treatments, may contain formaldehyde or formaldehyde-releasing agents to help smooth and straighten the hair. However, these treatments have raised health concerns due to potential formaldehyde exposure during application and heat styling.

4. **Eyelash Glue**: Formaldehyde-releasing agents may be present in some eyelash adhesives used for false eyelash application.

5. **Shampoos and Hair Products**: While less common, formaldehyde or formaldehyde-releasing agents may be used as preservatives in some shampoos, hair conditioners, and styling products.

6. **Body Washes and Cleansers**: Formaldehyde-releasing agents may be used in some body washes, cleansers, and shower gels to prevent microbial contamination.

7. **Cosmetic Wipes**: Some cosmetic wipes and towelettes may contain formaldehyde or formaldehyde-releasing agents as preservatives.

Some other common uses of formaldehyde include:

1. **Resins (A sticky substance)**: Formaldehyde is used in the manufacture of plywood, particleboard, medium-density fiberboard (MDF), and other wood products, as well as in adhesives, coatings, and laminates.

2. **Textiles**: Formaldehyde-based resins are used in the treatment of textiles to improve wrinkle resistance, shrink resistance, and colorfastness.

3. **Disinfectants**: Formaldehyde is used as a disinfectant and preservative in certain healthcare and laboratory settings.

4. **Biocides**: Formaldehyde-based biocides are used to control microbial growth in water-based systems, such as cooling towers and industrial process water.

5. **Embalming**: Formaldehyde is used in embalming fluids to preserve human, and animal remains for funeral or anatomical study purposes.

It's important to note that the use of formaldehyde and formaldehyde-releasing agents in cosmetics is regulated by health authorities in many countries, and there are limits on their concentrations in cosmetic products. Inhalation or ingestion of formaldehyde can cause irritation of the eyes, nose, and throat, as well as respiratory symptoms such as coughing and wheezing. Long-term exposure to formaldehyde has been associated with an increased risk of certain cancers, particularly nasopharyngeal cancer and leukemia.

Trigger 3/101 – Asbestos

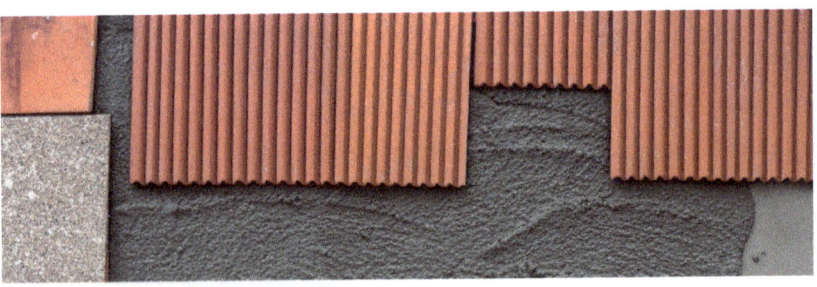

Report: 1st Report on Carcinogens
Carcinogen Category: environmental
Cancer Type(s): lung, mesothelioma, larynx(voice box), ovarian, stomach, pharynx(throat)

Unraveling the Origins: Exploring 101 Triggers of Cancer

Asbestos is a mineral fiber that was once widely used in construction and manufacturing due to its desirable properties such as heat resistance, strength, and insulating properties. It was commonly used in building materials like insulation, roofing, flooring, and in various automotive parts.

However, asbestos is now recognized as a serious health hazard because inhaling asbestos fibers can lead to various lung diseases, including asbestosis, lung cancer, and mesothelioma. Due to its carcinogenic properties, many countries have banned or heavily regulated the use of asbestos in recent decades.

Asbestos has been historically used in a wide range of products due to its heat resistance, strength, and insulating properties. Some common products that have historically contained asbestos include:

1. **Building materials**: Asbestos was commonly used in building materials such as insulation, roofing materials, ceiling tiles, floor tiles, and cement products.

2. **Automotive parts**: Asbestos was used in various automotive components including brake pads, brake linings, clutch facings, and gaskets.

3. **Textiles**: Asbestos fibers were used in textiles for their heat-resistant properties. Fire-resistant clothing, blankets, and gloves were some examples.

4. **Electrical insulation**: Asbestos was used in electrical insulation materials such as wire insulation, electrical cloth, and arc chutes in circuit breakers.

5. **Industrial applications**: Asbestos was used in various industrial applications including gaskets, packing materials for

pipes and machinery, and as a reinforcing agent in plastics and other materials.

6. **Consumer products**: Asbestos was also used in consumer products such as hair dryers, ironing board covers, and potholders for its heat resistance.

Due to its recognized health risks, the use of asbestos has declined significantly in many countries, and its use is now heavily regulated in various products and industries.

Trigger 4/101 – Haloacetic Acids

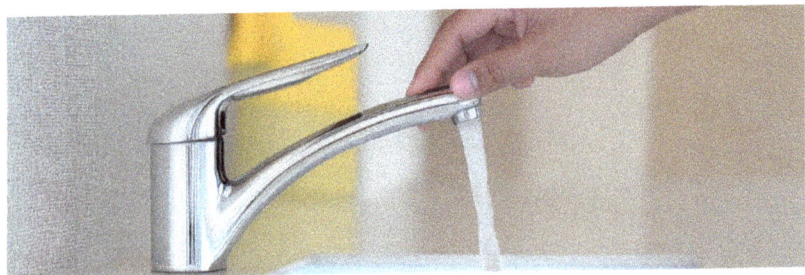

Report: 15th Report on Carcinogens
Category: chemical
Cancer Type(s): liver, kidney

Haloacetic acids (HAAs) are a group of organic chemical compounds that are formed as disinfection byproducts (DBPs) during the chlorination or chloramination of drinking water. They are derived from the reaction between chlorine or chloramines (disinfectants used in water treatment) and naturally occurring organic matter or other substances present in water sources.

Unraveling the Origins: Exploring 101 Triggers of Cancer

Exposure to haloacetic acids in drinking water has been associated with potential health risks. Studies have shown that long-term exposure to elevated levels of haloacetic acids may increase the risk of adverse health effects, including liver and kidney damage, reproductive and developmental effects, and an increased risk of cancer. The carcinogenicity of certain haloacetic acids, such as dichloroacetic acid (DCAA) and trichloroacetic acid (TCAA), has been demonstrated in animal studies, leading to their classification as possible human carcinogens by some regulatory agencies.

Due to their potential health risks, haloacetic acids are regulated by drinking water quality standards established by regulatory agencies, such as the U.S. Environmental Protection Agency (EPA). In the United States, the EPA has set maximum contaminant levels (MCLs) for total haloacetic acids (THAA), which include the sum of the concentrations of five specific haloacetic acids (MCAA, DCAA, TCAA, MBAA, and DBAA). Water utilities are required to monitor and control haloacetic acid levels in drinking water to ensure compliance with regulatory standards and protect public health.

The presence and levels of HAAs in drinking water can vary depending on factors such as the source water quality, the type and dosage of disinfectants used, the treatment processes employed, and the distribution system conditions. In general, HAAs are more likely to be found in drinking water supplies that rely on chlorination or chloramination for disinfection.

Overall, while chlorine and chloramines are important disinfectants used to ensure the safety of drinking water by controlling microbial contaminants, the formation of haloacetic acids as disinfection byproducts underscores the importance of balancing water disinfection goals with the need to minimize potentially harmful DBPs in drinking water supplies.

Trigger 5/101 – Dioxins

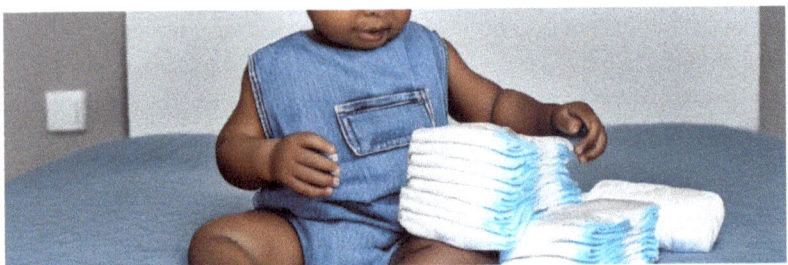

Report: 11th Report on Carcinogens
Category: chemical
Cancer Type(s): liver, sarcoma, non-hodgkin lymphoma, lung, prostate, breast, skin

Dioxins are a group of chemically related compounds that are persistent environmental pollutants. They belong to a larger class of substances known as persistent organic pollutants (POPs).

Dioxins can potentially be found in diapers, although efforts have been made to reduce their presence. Dioxins can be produced as byproducts during the bleaching process of the pulp used in diaper manufacturing. Chlorine bleaching, in particular, has been associated with dioxin formation. Some parents opt for organic or eco-friendly diaper brands that explicitly state they use TCF bleaching processes or other methods to avoid dioxins. These products often provide assurance that they are free from harmful chemicals, including dioxins.

Dioxins are primarily byproducts of industrial processes, including:

1. Incineration of waste (municipal, hazardous, and medical).

2. Chemical manufacturing processes, particularly those involving chlorine (e.g., herbicides and paper bleaching).

3. Combustion processes, such as forest fires and the burning of fossil fuels and wood.

4. Some natural processes like volcanic eruptions and forest fires.

Dioxins are highly stable and can persist in the environment for many years. They accumulate in the food chain, mainly in the fatty tissue of animals. Dioxins are classified as known human carcinogens. Long-term exposure can increase the risk of developing various cancers. Dioxins can affect reproductive health and development, leading to birth defects, reduced fertility, and developmental delays. Dioxins can suppress the immune system, reducing the ability to fight infections and diseases. Dioxins can interfere with hormonal systems, leading to a variety of health issues.

The primary route of human exposure to dioxins is through the consumption of animal fats (meat, dairy, fish, and eggs. People living near sources of dioxin pollution (industrial sites, waste incinerators) may have higher exposure levels.

Trigger 6/101 – Ultraviolet (UV) radiation

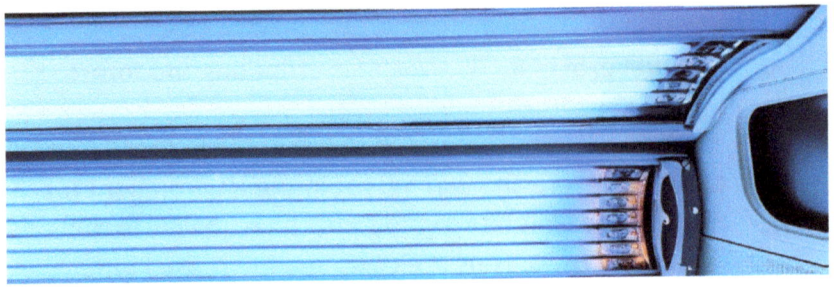

Report: 9th Report on Carcinogens
Carcinogen Category: physical
Cancer Type(s): skin, eye

Ultraviolet (UV) radiation is not a carcinogen in itself; rather, it is a form of electromagnetic radiation emitted by the sun and artificial sources such as tanning beds. UV radiation consists of three main types: UVA, UVB, and UVC.

UV radiation can cause damage to the DNA in skin cells, leading to mutations that can contribute to the development of skin cancer over time. Excessive exposure to UV radiation is a well-established risk factor for various types of skin cancer, including basal cell carcinoma, squamous cell carcinoma, and melanoma.

UV radiation exposure can also cause other adverse effects on the skin, such as premature aging (photoaging), sunburn, and the development of benign growths such as actinic keratoses.

Several studies have shown a clear link between tanning bed use and an increased risk of skin cancer, including melanoma, which is the deadliest form of skin cancer. Due to these risks, many health organizations, including the World Health Organization (WHO) and the American Academy of Dermatology (AAD), recommend avoiding the use of tanning beds altogether. Instead, they advise

Unraveling the Origins: Exploring 101 Triggers of Cancer

practicing sun safety measures, such as wearing protective clothing, seeking shade, and avoiding indoor tanning devices to reduce the risk of skin cancer.

Six artificial sources of broad-spectrum include:

1. incandescent lights
2. gas-discharge lamps
3. arc lamps
4. fluorescent lamps
5. metal halide lamps
6. electrodeless lamps

It's safe to say that the vast majority of the global population is exposed to UV radiation to some extent, with varying degrees of intensity.

Trigger 7/101 – Ionizing Radiation (X-rays, gamma rays)

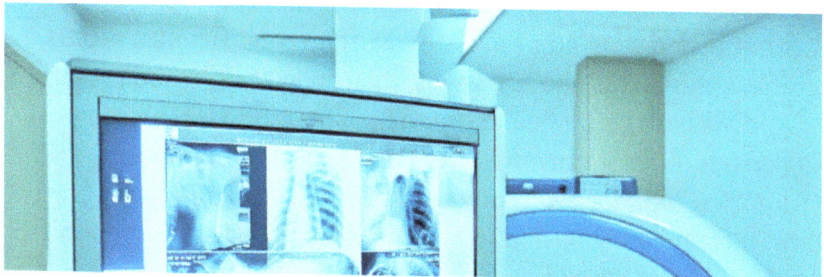

Report: 11th Report on Carcinogens
Carcinogen Category: physical
Cancer Type(s): leukemia, thyroid, breast, lung

X-ray machines operate by generating X-rays through the interaction of electrons with a metal anode, directing these X-rays

49

through the body, capturing the transmitted X-rays on a detector, and processing the resulting images for medical diagnosis.

An ion is an atom or molecule that has gained or lost one or more electrons, thus acquiring an electrical charge. Radiation refers to the emission and propagation of energy through space or a medium in the form of waves or particles. It can take various forms, including electromagnetic waves (such as light, radio waves, microwaves, X-rays, and gamma rays) and particles (such as alpha particles, beta particles, and neutrons).

Radiation can be categorized into two main types:

1. **Ionizing Radiation**: This type of radiation carries enough energy to remove tightly bound electrons from atoms, thereby ionizing them. Examples include X-rays, gamma rays, alpha particles, beta particles, and neutrons. Ionizing radiation can penetrate matter deeply and has the potential to cause damage to biological tissues and DNA, leading to health risks such as radiation sickness, cancer, and genetic mutations.

2. **Non-Ionizing Radiation**: Non-ionizing radiation carries less energy and does not have sufficient energy to ionize atoms. Examples include radio waves, microwaves, infrared radiation, and visible light. While non-ionizing radiation is generally considered less harmful to biological tissues compared to ionizing radiation, prolonged exposure to certain types (such as ultraviolet radiation from the sun) can still cause health effects, such as sunburn and skin cancer.

Exposure to high levels of ionizing radiation can be harmful to living organisms, damaging DNA and potentially leading to radiation sickness, cancer, or genetic mutations. Hence, it's carefully regulated and monitored in various applications to minimize risks to human health and the environment.

Unraveling the Origins: Exploring 101 Triggers of Cancer

Trigger 8/101 – Alcoholic Beverages

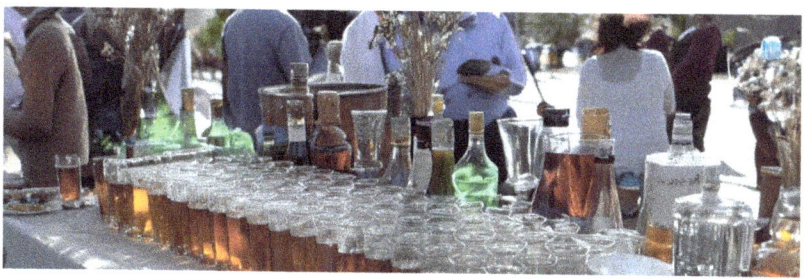

Report: 9th Report on Carcinogens
Carcinogen Category: chemical
Cancer Type(s): liver, breast, mouth, pharynx, larynx, esophagus

Ethanol and water are the primary components of most alcoholic beverages. According to standard serving sizes, the ethanol content in beer, wine, and spirits is comparable, typically ranging from 10 to 14 grams per serving.

There are several reasons why alcohol is associated with an increased risk of cancer:

1. **Metabolism**: When alcohol is consumed, it is metabolized in the body to acetaldehyde, a toxic and carcinogenic compound. Acetaldehyde can damage DNA and proteins, leading to mutations and promoting the growth of cancerous cells.

2. **Disruption of Cell Cycle**: Alcohol can interfere with the normal regulation of cell growth and division, disrupting the cell cycle. This disruption can contribute to the development of cancer by allowing abnormal cells to proliferate unchecked.

3. **Increased Estrogen Levels**: Alcohol can lead to increased levels of estrogen in the body, which has been linked to an elevated risk of breast and other hormone-related cancers.

4. **Oxidative Stress**: Alcohol consumption can induce oxidative stress in the body, leading to the production of reactive oxygen species (ROS) that can damage DNA and other cellular components, promoting carcinogenesis.

5. **Nutritional Deficiencies**: Chronic alcohol consumption can lead to nutritional deficiencies, such as deficiencies in folate, vitamin B6, and vitamin B12, which are important for DNA repair and maintenance. These deficiencies can further increase the risk of cancer.

6. **Immune System Suppression**: Alcohol consumption can weaken the immune system, impairing the body's ability to detect and destroy cancerous cells before they proliferate.

The risk of developing cancer increases with the amount and duration of alcohol consumption. Therefore, reducing or eliminating alcohol consumption can help lower the risk of alcohol-related cancers. Additionally, maintaining a healthy lifestyle, including a balanced diet and regular exercise, can also help mitigate the risk factors associated with alcohol consumption.

Unraveling the Origins: Exploring 101 Triggers of Cancer

Trigger 9/101 – Nitrosamines

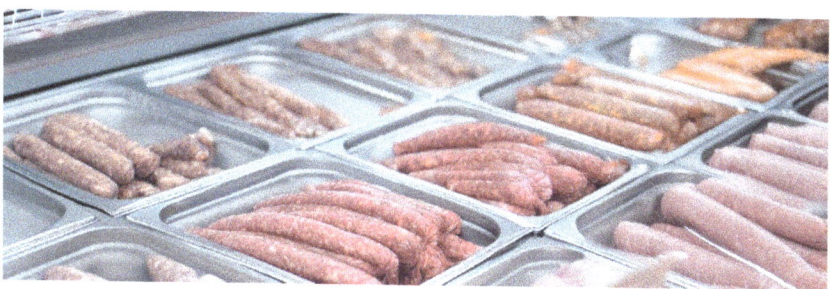

Report: 15th Report on Carcinogens
Carcinogen Category: chemical
Cancer Type(s): stomach, liver, brain, colon

Nitrosamines are formed through the reaction of nitrites with secondary amines or through the nitrosation of amines under acidic conditions. Nitrosamines are known to be potent carcinogens, meaning they can cause cancer in humans and animals.

Nitrosamines can be found in various environmental sources, including:

1. **Tobacco Smoke**: Tobacco smoke contains significant levels of nitrosamines, which are formed during the curing process of tobacco leaves and during the combustion of tobacco products. Nitrosamines in tobacco smoke are strongly associated with the development of lung cancer and other tobacco-related cancers.

2. **Processed Meats**: Nitrosamines can form in processed meats (such as bacon, sausage, and ham) during curing, smoking, or cooking, especially when nitrite-containing agents are used. Consuming processed meats has been linked to an increased

risk of colorectal and stomach cancer.

3. **Occupational Exposure**: Certain industries, such as rubber manufacturing, pesticide production, and metalworking, may involve processes that produce nitrosamines as byproducts. Workers in these industries may be exposed to nitrosamines through inhalation or skin contact.

4. **Food and Beverages**: Nitrosamines can form in foods and beverages, particularly under conditions of high temperature and low pH (acidity). For example, nitrosamines can form in beer during brewing or in pickled or fermented foods.

5. **Cosmetics**: As of 1980, the U.S. Food and Drug Administration had analyzed over 300 cosmetic products and found that over 40% were contaminated with N-nitrosodiethanolamine. It was detected in facial cosmetics, lotions, soaps and in shampoos. Nitrosamines are formed within these products by reactions of precursors (nitrosating agents and primary or secondary amines) or are introduced using contaminated raw materials.

Strategies for reducing nitrosamine exposure include controlling processing conditions in food production, limiting the use of nitrite-containing additives, and implementing tobacco control measures to reduce smoking-related exposure.

Unraveling the Origins: Exploring 101 Triggers of Cancer

Trigger 10/101 – Vinyl Chloride

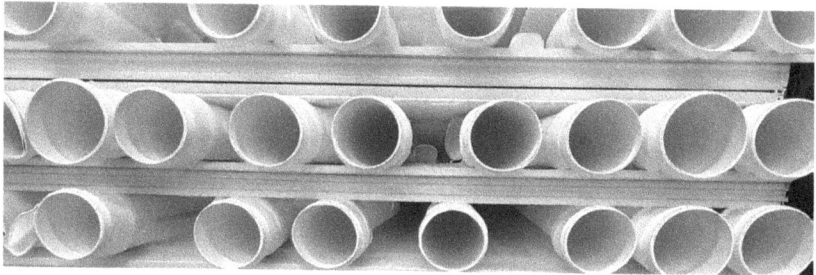

Report: 1st Report on Carcinogens
Carcinogen Category: chemical
Cancer Type(s): liver, brain, lung, lymphatic

Vinyl chloride is an important industrial chemical used primarily in the production of polyvinyl chloride (PVC), a widely used plastic material.

Vinyl chloride is produced through the chemical reaction of ethylene gas with chlorine gas in a process called chlorination. The resulting vinyl chloride can then be polymerized to form PVC resin, which is further processed into various products such as pipes, fittings, siding, window frames, and medical devices.

While PVC itself is not considered toxic, vinyl chloride, the precursor used to make PVC, is known to be highly toxic and carcinogenic. Prolonged or high-level exposure to vinyl chloride can have serious health effects, including:

1. **Cancer**: Vinyl chloride is classified as a Group 1 carcinogen by the International Agency for Research on Cancer (IARC), meaning it is known to cause cancer in humans. Long-term exposure to vinyl chloride has been linked to an increased risk of liver cancer, particularly angiosarcoma of the liver, as well as lung cancer and some other cancers.

2. **Central Nervous System Effects**: Acute exposure to high levels of vinyl chloride can cause symptoms such as dizziness, drowsiness, and headaches. In severe cases, it can lead to unconsciousness and death due to respiratory failure.

3. **Liver Damage**: Vinyl chloride is primarily metabolized in the liver. Chronic exposure to vinyl chloride can lead to liver damage, including fatty liver, liver fibrosis, and cirrhosis.

In the past, vinyl chloride was detected in various foods and beverages that were packaged in materials made of PVC; however, U.S. FDA regulations have essentially eliminated this route of exposure. Some water pipes are made using PVC. PVC is commonly used for plumbing because it is durable, resistant to corrosion, and relatively inexpensive.

Due to its toxic and carcinogenic properties, strict regulations govern the handling, storage, and disposal of vinyl chloride in industrial settings. People who work in industries that produce or use vinyl chloride, such as plastics manufacturing, are at higher risk. They may be exposed through inhalation of vinyl chloride gas or skin contact with liquid vinyl chloride.

Unraveling the Origins: Exploring 101 Triggers of Cancer

Trigger 11/101 – Human Papillomavirus (HPV)

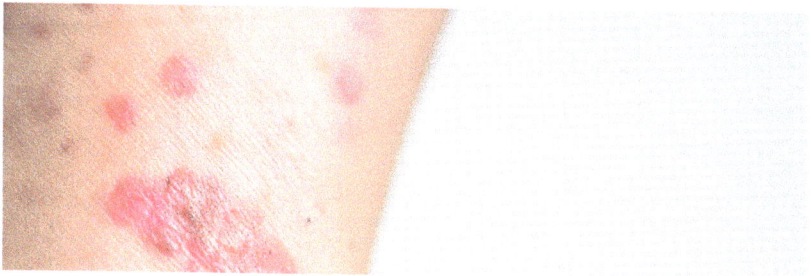

Report: 13th Report on Carcinogens
Carcinogen Category: biological
Cancer Type(s): cervical, oral, head and neck

Human papillomavirus (HPV) is considered a carcinogen because certain types of HPV infections have been conclusively linked to the development of several types of cancer. HPV is a group of viruses that infect the skin and mucous membranes of humans. There are over 100 different types of HPV, some of which are categorized as high-risk types due to their association with cancer. Here's why HPV is considered a carcinogen:

1. **Integration into Host DNA**: High-risk HPV types, particularly HPV types 16 and 18, have the ability to integrate their genetic material into the DNA of infected cells. This integration disrupts normal cellular processes, leading to uncontrolled cell growth and potentially the development of cancer.

2. **Inactivation of Tumor Suppressors**: HPV oncoproteins, such as E6 and E7, produced by high-risk HPV types, can inactivate tumor suppressor genes, which normally help regulate cell growth and prevent the development of cancer. Inactivation of these genes allows infected cells to proliferate uncontrollably, increasing the risk of cancer.

3. **Induction of Genomic Instability**: HPV infection can induce genomic instability in infected cells, leading to the accumulation of genetic mutations. This genomic instability can promote the development of cancer by allowing cells to acquire additional mutations that drive tumor formation and progression.

4. **Inflammation and Immune Suppression**: Chronic inflammation and immune suppression associated with persistent HPV infection can create a microenvironment that promotes cancer development. Inflammation can lead to tissue damage and stimulate cell proliferation, while immune suppression reduces the ability of the immune system to detect and eliminate cancerous cells.

HPV is most associated with cervical cancer, but it can also cause other types of cancer, including anal cancer, penile cancer, vaginal cancer, vulvar cancer, and oropharyngeal cancer (cancers of the throat, tongue, and tonsils).

Strategies for reducing the effects of having this virus include proper diet and nutrition, natural antiviral herbs, and detoxifying the body of heavy metals.

Unraveling the Origins: Exploring 101 Triggers of Cancer

Trigger 12/101 – Hepatitis B Virus

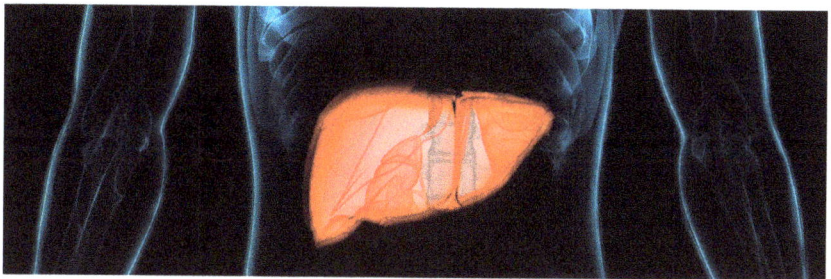

Report: 9th Report on Carcinogens
Carcinogen Category: biological
Cancer Type(s): liver

Hepatitis B virus (HBV) is considered a carcinogen because chronic infection with HBV can lead to the development of liver cancer, also known as hepatocellular carcinoma (HCC). Here's why HBV is associated with carcinogenicity:

1. **Integration of Viral DNA**: Chronic HBV infection can lead to the integration of viral DNA into the host cell's genome. This integration can disrupt cellular processes, including those involved in cell growth regulation, and promote the development of cancer.

2. **Chronic Hepatitis and Liver Inflammation**: HBV infection often results in chronic hepatitis, characterized by persistent inflammation of the liver. Chronic inflammation can lead to tissue damage, regeneration, and the formation of fibrosis and cirrhosis, which are precursors to liver cancer.

3. **Production of Viral Proteins**: HBV encodes several viral proteins, including the hepatitis B virus X protein (HBx). These proteins can interfere with cellular processes such as DNA repair, apoptosis (programmed cell death), and cell cycle regulation, promoting cell proliferation and contributing to the

development of cancer.

4. **Immune-mediated Mechanisms**: Chronic HBV infection can lead to immune dysregulation and suppression, allowing infected cells to evade immune surveillance and persist in the liver. This immune evasion can contribute to the progression of liver disease and the development of cancer.

5. **Synergistic Effects with Other Carcinogens**: Chronic HBV infection can synergize with other risk factors for liver cancer, such as chronic hepatitis C virus (HCV) infection, alcohol consumption, aflatoxin exposure, and metabolic disorders like non-alcoholic fatty liver disease (NAFLD). These synergistic effects can further increase the risk of liver cancer in individuals with chronic HBV infection.

It's important to note that not all individuals with chronic HBV infection develop liver cancer. Factors such as the duration of infection, viral load, host genetic factors, and environmental exposures play a role in determining the risk of cancer development. Regular screening for liver cancer in individuals with chronic HBV infection is important for early detection and treatment.

Unraveling the Origins: Exploring 101 Triggers of Cancer

Trigger 13/101 – Helicobacter Pylori

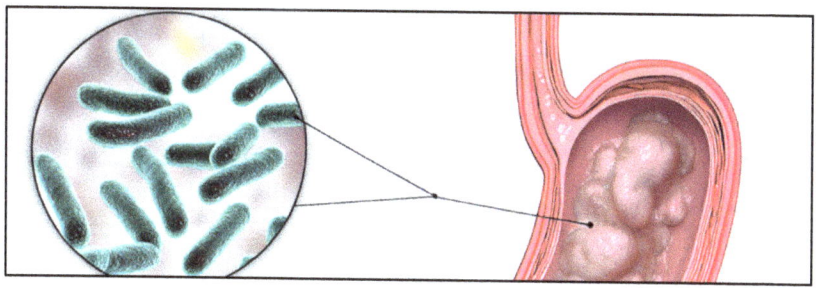

Report: 15th Report on Carcinogens
Carcinogen Category: biological
Cancer Type(s): stomach, gastric MALT lymphoma

Helicobacter pylori (H. pylori) is a bacterium that infects the stomach lining and is a major risk factor for the development of certain types of stomach cancer, particularly non-cardia gastric adenocarcinoma and gastric mucosa-associated lymphoid tissue (MALT) lymphoma. Here's why H. pylori is considered a carcinogen:

1. **Chronic Gastritis and Inflammation**: H. pylori infection triggers a chronic inflammatory response in the stomach lining, leading to persistent gastritis. Chronic inflammation can damage the gastric epithelium, promote tissue repair and regeneration, and create an environment conducive to carcinogenesis.

2. **Production of Toxins**: H. pylori produce various virulence factors, including cytotoxin-associated gene A (CagA) and vacuolating cytotoxin A (VacA), which can directly damage gastric epithelial cells and promote cellular proliferation. These toxins can disrupt cellular signaling pathways, interfere with DNA repair mechanisms, and induce genetic instability,

contributing to the development of cancer.

3. **Induction of DNA Damage**: H. pylori infection can lead to the generation of reactive oxygen and nitrogen species (ROS/RNS) in the stomach lining. These reactive molecules can cause oxidative DNA damage, including DNA strand breaks, base modifications, and DNA cross-linking, which can lead to genetic mutations and promote carcinogenesis.

4. **Alteration of Host Cell Signaling**: H. pylori infection can alter host cell signaling pathways involved in cell proliferation, apoptosis (programmed cell death), and immune response. Dysregulation of these signaling pathways can promote cell survival and proliferation and inhibit apoptosis, allowing damaged cells to accumulate and progress towards cancer.

5. **Interaction with Host Immune System**: H. pylori has evolved mechanisms to evade host immune responses, allowing it to establish chronic infection and persist in the stomach lining for years to decades. Chronic immune stimulation and dysregulation associated with H. pylori infection can contribute to tissue damage, inflammation, and carcinogenesis.

While H. pylori infection is a major risk factor for stomach cancer, not all individuals infected with H. pylori develop cancer. Factors such as bacterial strain virulence, host genetic susceptibility, environmental factors (such as diet and smoking), and co-infections with other pathogens can influence the risk of cancer development in individuals with H. pylori infection.

Unraveling the Origins: Exploring 101 Triggers of Cancer

Trigger 14/101 – Aflatoxins

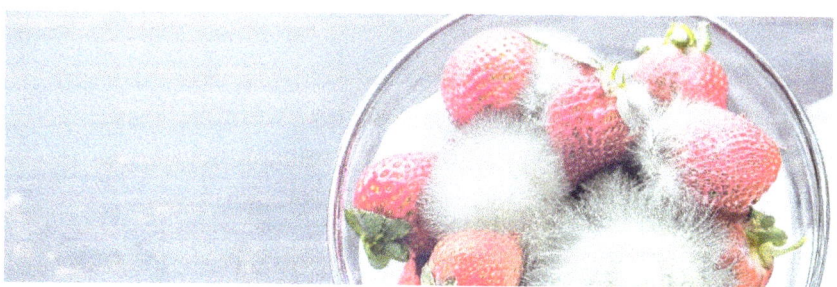

Report: 1st Report on Carcinogens
Carcinogen Category: biological
Cancer Type(s): liver, colon, bone, gallbladder, pancreas

Aflatoxins are potent carcinogenic toxins produced by certain molds, primarily Aspergillus flavus and Aspergillus parasiticus, which commonly contaminate food crops such as peanuts, corn, cottonseed, and tree nuts. Here's why aflatoxins are considered carcinogens:

1. **DNA Damage**: Aflatoxins can bind to DNA in cells, leading to the formation of DNA adducts. These adducts can cause mutations in critical genes involved in cell cycle regulation, DNA repair, and apoptosis (programmed cell death). Mutations induced by aflatoxins can promote the development of cancer.

2. **Liver Toxicity**: Aflatoxins are primarily metabolized in the liver by enzymes such as cytochrome P450. During metabolism, aflatoxins can produce reactive metabolites that cause oxidative stress, mitochondrial dysfunction, and lipid peroxidation, leading to liver cell damage and inflammation. Chronic exposure to aflatoxins can result in liver cirrhosis and hepatocellular carcinoma (HCC), a type of liver cancer.

3. **Immunosuppression**: Aflatoxin exposure can suppress the immune system, impairing the body's ability to detect and eliminate cancerous cells. A compromised immune response allows tumor cells to proliferate unchecked, contributing to the development and progression of cancer.

4. **Synergistic Effects with Hepatitis B Virus (HBV)**: Aflatoxin exposure has been shown to synergize with chronic infection with hepatitis B virus (HBV) to increase the risk of liver cancer. Chronic HBV infection can enhance the carcinogenic effects of aflatoxins by promoting liver inflammation, DNA damage, and cell proliferation.

5. **Epigenetic Changes**: Aflatoxins can induce epigenetic changes in cells, altering patterns of gene expression without changing the underlying DNA sequence. These epigenetic changes can affect the expression of genes involved in cell growth regulation, apoptosis, and DNA repair, promoting carcinogenesis.

Aflatoxins are one of the most potent naturally occurring carcinogens known, and exposure to even low levels of aflatoxins over a long period can increase the risk of cancer. Strategies to reduce aflatoxin exposure include implementing good agricultural practices to prevent mold growth in crops, proper storage and handling of food to minimize aflatoxin contamination, and regular monitoring and testing of food products for aflatoxin levels. Additionally, dietary interventions and nutritional supplements may help mitigate the adverse effects of aflatoxin exposure on human health.

Unraveling the Origins: Exploring 101 Triggers of Cancer

Trigger 15/101 – Benzidine

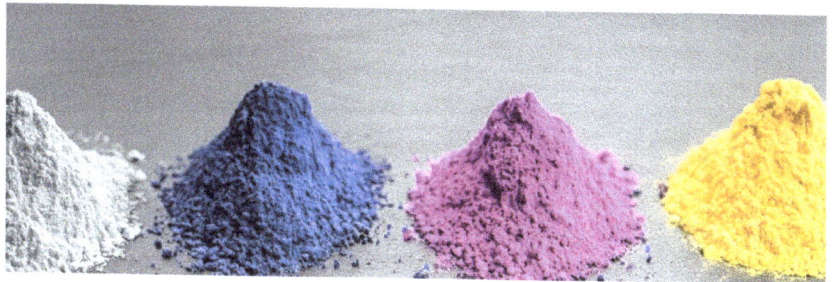

Report: 1st Report on Carcinogens
Carcinogen Category: chemical
Cancer Type(s): bladder, kidney, liver

Benzidine is a highly toxic and carcinogenic compound that was once widely used in the production of dyes, particularly azo dyes, and pigments. Azo dyes are a class of synthetic dyes used in many common consumer products such as clothing, leather, carpets and other textiles. These dyes are also found in food and cosmetics. Benzidine-based dyes were mainly utilized for coloring textiles, leather, and paper products, as well as in the petroleum, rubber, plastics, wood, soap, fur, and hair-dye industries. Approximately 40% of these dyes were used in paper coloring, 25% in textile coloring, 15% in leather coloring, and the remaining 20% for various other applications.

Here's why benzidine is considered a carcinogen:

1. **DNA Damage**: Benzidine is metabolized in the body to form reactive intermediates that can bind to DNA, leading to the formation of DNA adducts. These adducts can cause mutations in critical genes involved in cell cycle regulation, DNA repair, and apoptosis (programmed cell death). Mutations induced by benzidine can promote the development of cancer.

2. **Bladder Carcinogenesis**: Chronic exposure to benzidine has been strongly linked to the development of bladder cancer. After absorption in the body, benzidine is primarily excreted in the urine. In the bladder, benzidine and its metabolites can come into direct contact with the bladder epithelium, leading to DNA damage, cell proliferation, and the formation of pre-cancerous and cancerous lesions.

3. **Metabolic Activation**: Benzidine undergoes metabolic activation by enzymes leading to the formation of reactive metabolites that can damage DNA and other cellular components. The metabolic activation of benzidine is thought to play a key role in its carcinogenicity.

Overall, benzidine is a potent carcinogen that poses significant health risks to individuals exposed to it, particularly through occupational routes. Efforts to minimize exposure to benzidine and benzidine-based compounds are essential for preventing the associated health effects, particularly bladder cancer.

Unraveling the Origins: Exploring 101 Triggers of Cancer

Trigger 16/101 – Cadmium (Smelting)

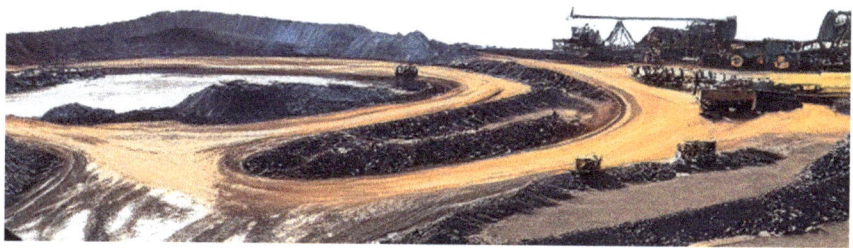

Report: 9th Report on Carcinogens
Carcinogen Category: environment
Cancer Type(s): lung, lymphoma, adrenal, liver, testicular, leukemia

Cadmium is a naturally occurring element found in the Earth's crust at relatively low concentrations. It is often associated with zinc, lead, and copper ores, and is typically found in mineral deposits such as zinc sulfide (sphalerite), lead sulfide (galena), and copper sulfide (chalcopyrite). Smelting is the extraction of metal from its ore by a process involving heating and melting.

The primary sources of cadmium include:

1. **Mining and Smelting**: Cadmium is commonly co-extracted during the mining and smelting of zinc, lead, and copper ores. It is often present in ores as an impurity and is released into the environment during the extraction and processing of these metals.

2. **Industrial Processes**: Cadmium is used in industrial processes and products, including the production of batteries, pigments, coatings, plastics, and alloys. Industrial activities such as metal plating, electroplating, welding, and manufacturing can

release cadmium into the air, water, and soil.

3. **Tobacco Smoke**: Tobacco plants are known to absorb cadmium from soil, and cadmium levels in tobacco leaves can be elevated in areas with cadmium-rich soils. Smoking tobacco products exposes individuals to cadmium through inhalation of cadmium-containing tobacco smoke.

4. **Fertilizers and Phosphate Mining**: Some fertilizers and phosphate-containing soil amendments may contain cadmium as a contaminant. Cadmium can be present in phosphate rock deposits, and its use in fertilizers can lead to cadmium accumulation in agricultural soils.

5. **Waste Disposal Sites**: Cadmium-containing waste from industrial processes, electronic devices, batteries, and consumer products can be disposed of in landfills or dumped into water bodies, leading to contamination of soil and water.

Due to its widespread use in various industries and products, cadmium can be found in air, water, soil, and food at varying concentrations. Human activities such as mining, manufacturing, and waste disposal can contribute to environmental cadmium contamination. Efforts to monitor and regulate cadmium emissions, minimize exposure in occupational settings, and reduce environmental contamination are important for protecting public health and the environment.

Unraveling the Origins: Exploring 101 Triggers of Cancer

Trigger 17/101 – Chromium Hexavalent

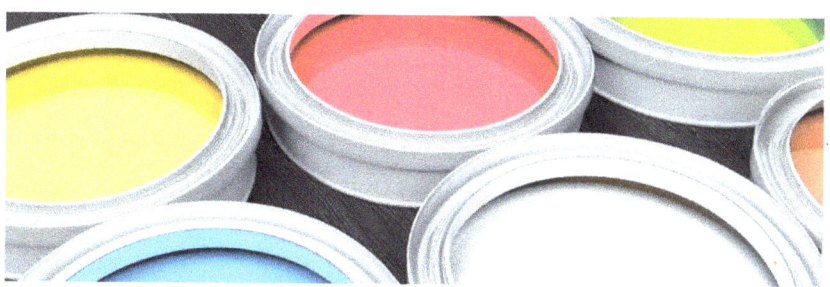

Report: 1st Report on Carcinogens
Carcinogen Category: chemical
Cancer Type(s): lung, lymphoma, adrenal, liver, testicular, leukemia

Hexavalent chromium is highly toxic and carcinogenic form of chromium. Hexavalent chromium compounds are often produced as industrial byproducts and are used in various industrial processes, including:

1. **Metal Plating**: Hexavalent chromium is used in chrome plating to provide a decorative and corrosion-resistant coating on metal surfaces, such as automotive parts, appliances, and furniture.

2. **Paints and Coatings**: Hexavalent chromium compounds are used as pigments and colorants in paints, inks, and coatings, particularly in the production of yellow, orange, and red pigments.

3. **Tanneries and Leather Production**: Hexavalent chromium is used in leather tanning processes to help stabilize collagen fibers and improve the quality and durability of leather products.

4. **Electronics Manufacturing**: Hexavalent chromium is used in the production of electronic components, such as printed circuit boards and semiconductors, as a corrosion inhibitor and solder flux.

5. **Wood Preservation**: Hexavalent chromium compounds have been used in wood preservation treatments to protect against decay and insect damage, although their use has been largely phased out due to environmental concerns.

Hexavalent chromium is highly soluble in water and can easily enter the environment through industrial discharge, runoff from contaminated sites, and improper disposal practices. Inhalation of hexavalent chromium-containing dusts or fumes and ingestion of contaminated food or water are common routes of human exposure.

Exposure to hexavalent chromium can have serious health effects, including irritation and damage to the respiratory system, skin, and eyes. Long-term exposure to hexavalent chromium has been associated with an increased risk of lung cancer, nasal and sinus cancer, and other respiratory cancers. Due to its toxicity and carcinogenicity, regulations and safety measures are in place to minimize human exposure to hexavalent chromium in occupational and environmental settings.

Unraveling the Origins: Exploring 101 Triggers of Cancer

Trigger 18/101 – Ethylene Oxide

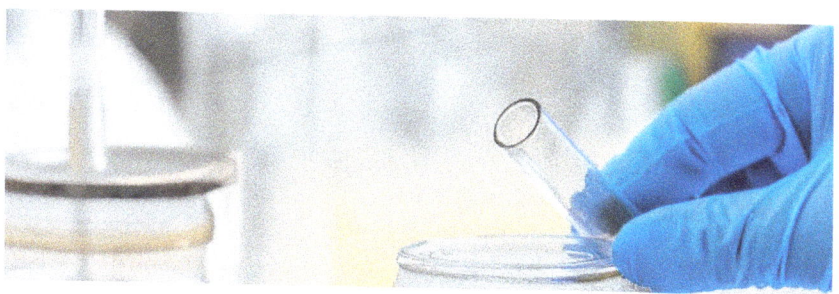

Report: 4th Report on Carcinogens
Carcinogen Category: chemical
Cancer Type(s): lung, breast, uterus, brain

Ethylene oxide (EO) is a highly reactive and flammable gas at room temperature. It is a versatile chemical compound used in various industrial applications, including:

1. **Sterilization**: Ethylene oxide is widely used for the sterilization of medical equipment and supplies, particularly those that are heat-sensitive and cannot be sterilized by steam or high-temperature methods. Ethylene oxide sterilization is effective against a wide range of microorganisms, including bacteria, viruses, fungi, and spores.

2. **Chemical Synthesis**: Ethylene oxide serves as a precursor in the production of several important chemicals, including ethylene glycol, which is used in the manufacture of polyester fibers, polyethylene terephthalate (PET) plastics, antifreeze, and other industrial products. Ethylene oxide is also used in the synthesis of surfactants, detergents, glycol ethers, and various organic compounds.

3. **Fumigation and Pest Control**: Ethylene oxide is used as a fumigant and insecticide for the treatment of stored grains,

spices, and other agricultural products to control pests and pathogens. It penetrates packaging materials and kills insects, larvae, and microorganisms present in the treated commodities.

4. **Chemical Intermediate**: Ethylene oxide serves as a versatile chemical intermediate in the production of other compounds which are used in the manufacture of cosmetics, personal care products, pharmaceuticals, and industrial chemicals.

While ethylene oxide has many industrial uses, it is also classified as a carcinogen by the International Agency for Research on Cancer (IARC) due to its association with an increased risk of cancer, particularly leukemia and lymphoma, as well as respiratory and gastrointestinal cancers. Long-term occupational exposure to ethylene oxide has been linked to an elevated risk of cancer among workers in industries such as chemical manufacturing, sterilization facilities, and agricultural fumigation.

Trigger 19/101 – Lead

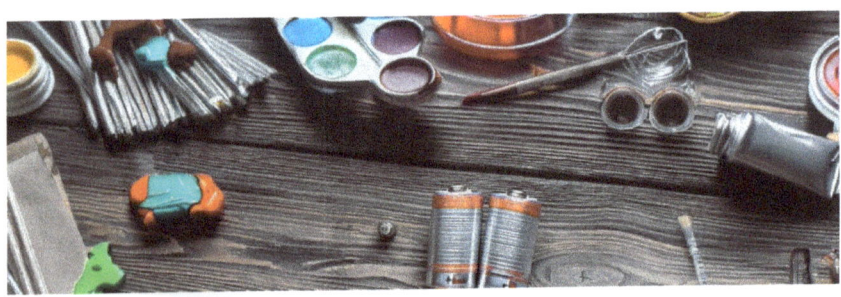

Report: 11th Report on Carcinogens
Carcinogen Category: chemical
Cancer Type(s): lung, stomach, kidney, bladder, brain, liver, colon

Unraveling the Origins: Exploring 101 Triggers of Cancer

Lead has been widely used in various products and industries due to its desirable properties, such as durability, malleability, and resistance to corrosion. However, due to its toxicity, its use in many consumer products has been restricted or banned in many countries. Nevertheless, lead can still be found in certain products, particularly in older items or those manufactured in regions with less stringent regulations. Here are some products that may contain lead:

1. **Paint**: Lead-based paint was commonly used in homes, buildings, and consumer products until its ban in many countries in the late 20th century. However, older homes and buildings may still have lead-based paint on walls, doors, windows, and furniture. Ingestion or inhalation of lead dust from deteriorating lead-based paint can pose health risks, particularly to children.

2. **Water Pipes and Plumbing Fixtures**: Lead can leach into drinking water from lead-containing pipes, solder, and plumbing fixtures, particularly in older homes and buildings. Lead contamination of drinking water can occur due to corrosion of lead pipes or solder joints, especially in areas with acidic water or low mineral content.

3. **Toys and Children's Products**: Lead has been used in the production of toys, jewelry, and other children's products as a pigment, stabilizer, or weight additive. While regulations limit the use of lead in children's products, imported items may still contain lead, particularly those manufactured in countries with lax regulations.

4. **Ceramics and Pottery**: Lead glazes have been used in the production of ceramics, pottery, and porcelain to create shiny or colorful finishes. Lead can leach from these products into food and beverages, especially acidic or hot items, posing a

risk of lead exposure.

5. **Imported Cosmetics and Traditional Remedies**: Certain cosmetics, especially those imported from countries with less stringent regulations, may contain lead as a contaminant or pigment. Lead has also been found in some traditional remedies and folk medicines used in certain cultures.

6. **Lead-Acid Batteries**: Lead-acid batteries, commonly used in vehicles, backup power systems, and industrial applications, contain lead in the form of lead plates and lead oxide. Improper handling or disposal of lead-acid batteries can lead to environmental contamination.

7. **Ammunition and Firearms**: Lead has historically been used in ammunition, bullets, and firearm components, although efforts have been made to develop lead-free alternatives due to environmental concerns.

It's important to note that exposure to lead can pose serious health risks, particularly to children, pregnant women, and fetuses. Efforts to minimize lead exposure include regular testing for lead in homes, schools, and drinking water, as well as strict regulation of lead in consumer products and industrial processes

Unraveling the Origins: Exploring 101 Triggers of Cancer

Trigger 20/101 – Polycyclic Aromatic Hydrocarbon

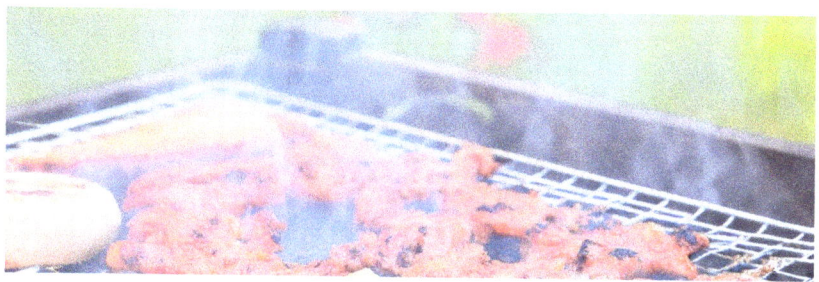

Report: 5th Report on Carcinogens
Carcinogen Category: chemical
Cancer Type(s): lung, stomach, skin, breast,

Polycyclic aromatic hydrocarbons (PAHs) are widespread environmental pollutants found in various products and materials. While PAHs are not intentionally added to products, they can be formed during the incomplete combustion of organic materials and are often present as contaminants in certain products.

Here are some examples of products that may contain PAHs:

1. **Smoked and Grilled Foods**: PAHs can form when foods, especially meats, are cooked at high temperatures through processes such as grilling, smoking, or charbroiling. The smoke from these cooking methods can deposit PAHs onto the surface of the food.

2. **Charcoal-Grilled Foods**: Foods cooked over charcoal or wood-fired grills can contain PAHs due to the incomplete combustion of the fuel, which generates PAH-containing smoke that can come into contact with the food.

3. **Barbecue and Smoked Meats**: Meats that have been smoked or barbecued are likely to contain PAHs due to the exposure

to smoke during the cooking process. This includes items like smoked sausages, smoked salmon, and barbecue ribs.

4. **Charred Foods**: Foods that are charred or blackened, such as grilled vegetables or charred bread, may contain higher levels of PAHs due to the formation of charred or burnt surfaces during cooking.

5. **Smoked Fish and Seafood**: Smoked fish and seafood products, such as smoked salmon or smoked mackerel, may contain PAHs due to the smoking process used for preservation and flavor enhancement.

6. **Creosote-Treated Wood Products**: Wood products treated with creosote, a preservative containing PAHs, may release PAHs into the environment over time. These products include railroad ties, utility poles, fencing, and outdoor decking.

7. **Coal-Tar Sealants**: Coal-tar-based sealants used for asphalt paving, driveway sealcoating, and parking lot maintenance can contain high levels of PAHs. These sealants can release PAHs into the air, soil, and water, contributing to environmental contamination.

8. **Secondhand Tobacco Smoke**: Tobacco smoke contains numerous chemicals, including PAHs, which are formed during the combustion of tobacco. Secondhand smoke exposure can result in inhalation and dermal contact with PAHs.

PAHs are widespread environmental pollutants found in air, water, soil, sediment, and food. It's important to note that exposure to PAHs from these products can vary depending on factors such as cooking methods, product composition, and environmental conditions. Efforts to minimize PAH exposure include choosing cooking methods that produce less smoke,

Unraveling the Origins: Exploring 101 Triggers of Cancer

avoiding charred or overcooked foods, and using alternative materials for outdoor structures and surfaces that come into contact with food. Additionally, regulations and guidelines may be in place to limit the use of certain PAH-containing products and to mitigate environmental contamination.

Trigger 21/101 – Radon

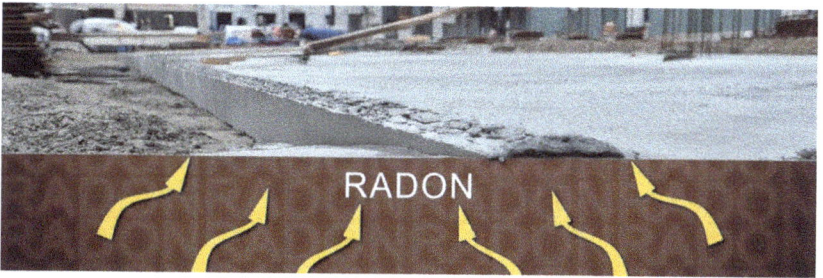

Report: 7th Report on Carcinogens
Carcinogen Category: environmental
Cancer Type(s): lung, leukemia, thyroid, breast

Radon is a naturally occurring radioactive gas that is colorless, odorless, and tasteless. It is formed by the radioactive decay of uranium, which is present in small amounts in soil, rock, and groundwater. Radon is a significant health hazard when it accumulates indoors, particularly in enclosed spaces such as homes and buildings.

Here are some key points about radon:

1. **Radioactivity**: Radon is radioactive and emits alpha particles as it decays. These alpha particles can damage lung tissue when inhaled, increasing the risk of lung cancer. Radon is the second leading cause of lung cancer after smoking and is

responsible for thousands of lung cancer deaths each year worldwide.

2. **Entry into Buildings**: Radon can enter buildings through cracks in the foundation, gaps around pipes and cables, and other openings in the building envelope. Once inside, radon can accumulate to high concentrations, especially in poorly ventilated or tightly sealed spaces.

3. **Geographical Variation**: Radon levels can vary widely depending on geographical location, soil composition, and building characteristics. Certain regions, particularly those with high levels of uranium in the underlying soil and rock, may have higher radon levels than others.

4. **Health Effects**: Long-term exposure to high levels of radon increases the risk of lung cancer, especially in smokers. Radon gas decays into radioactive particles that can become trapped in the lungs, where they emit radiation and damage lung tissue over time. Radon-related lung cancer typically develops over many years of exposure.

5. **Testing and Mitigation**: Radon testing is the only way to determine if a building has elevated radon levels. Testing kits are available for purchase, and professional radon testing services are also available. If elevated radon levels are detected, mitigation measures such as sealing cracks in the foundation, improving ventilation, and installing radon mitigation systems can reduce radon levels and minimize health risks.

6. **Regulations and Guidelines**: Many countries have established regulations and guidelines for radon exposure in homes and workplaces. These regulations may include permissible radon concentration levels, requirements for radon testing and

mitigation in certain types of buildings, and public awareness and education programs about radon risks and prevention.

Overall, radon is a significant environmental health concern that requires attention and proactive measures to mitigate exposure and protect public health. Radon is not intentionally added to products, nor is it used in manufacturing processes. Instead, radon is a naturally occurring radioactive gas that can be found in certain geological formations, soil, water, and building materials. Therefore, products themselves do not contain radon, but radon can enter indoor environments through various pathways and accumulate to high concentrations.

Trigger 22/101 – Anabolic Steroids

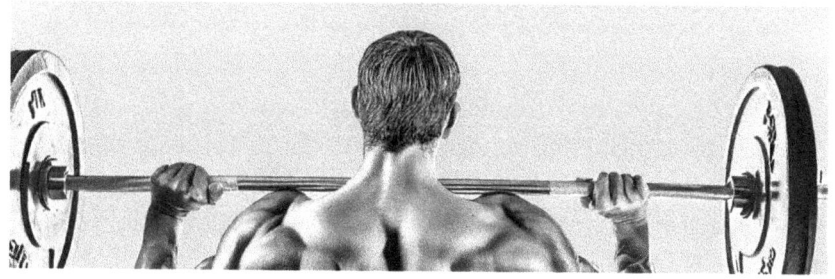

Report: NIH - PMC5922407
Carcinogen Category: chemical
Cancer Type(s): prostate, breast, testicular

Anabolic steroids, also known as anabolic-androgenic steroids (AAS), are synthetic variations of the male sex hormone testosterone. They are classified as Schedule III controlled substances in the United States due to their potential for abuse and misuse. Anabolic steroids are primarily used to promote muscle growth, enhance athletic performance, and improve physical appearance.

Here are some key points about anabolic steroids:

1. **Muscle Growth**: Anabolic steroids promote muscle growth by increasing protein synthesis and reducing protein breakdown in muscle cells. This leads to an increase in muscle mass, strength, and endurance.

2. **Performance Enhancement**: Athletes and bodybuilders may use anabolic steroids to improve athletic performance, speed up recovery from intense workouts, and gain a competitive edge. Some athletes may also use steroids to enhance their physical appearance by reducing body fat and increasing muscle definition.

3. **Medical Uses**: Anabolic steroids have legitimate medical uses and are prescribed to treat conditions such as delayed puberty, hormonal imbalances, muscle wasting diseases (e.g., AIDS-related wasting syndrome), and certain types of anemia. They may also be used to promote weight gain and muscle recovery in patients undergoing surgery or recovering from severe injuries.

4. **Administration**: Anabolic steroids can be administered orally, injected intramuscularly, or applied topically as creams or gels. Different formulations and dosing regimens may be used depending on the intended medical or performance-enhancing purpose.

5. **Side Effects**: While anabolic steroids can have beneficial effects on muscle growth and performance, they also carry significant risks and side effects. Common side effects of anabolic steroid use include acne, oily skin, hair loss, liver

damage, cardiovascular problems (e.g., high blood pressure, heart disease), hormonal imbalances, infertility, and mood disturbances (e.g., aggression, depression).

6. **Addiction and Dependence**: Anabolic steroid abuse can lead to psychological dependence and addiction, characterized by compulsive drug-seeking behavior, tolerance (requiring higher doses to achieve the desired effects), and withdrawal symptoms when discontinuing use.

7. **Legality**: The use, possession, and distribution of anabolic steroids without a prescription are illegal in many countries, including the United States. Violators may face legal consequences, including fines and imprisonment.

Due to the potential for abuse and the serious health risks associated with anabolic steroid use, their use should be limited to legitimate medical purposes under the supervision of a qualified healthcare professional. Individuals considering the use of anabolic steroids for performance enhancement should be aware of the potential risks and seek guidance from a healthcare provider.

The misuse or abuse of anabolic steroids may indirectly increase the risk of certain cancers due to several factors:

1. **Hormonal Imbalance**: Anabolic steroids disrupt the body's natural hormone balance, particularly by increasing levels of testosterone and other androgens. Prolonged exposure to high levels of androgens can lead to hormonal imbalances, which may contribute to the development of hormone-related cancers such as prostate cancer in men and breast cancer in women.

2. **Liver Toxicity**: Anabolic steroids can be hepatotoxic, meaning they can cause damage to the liver. Prolonged use of oral anabolic steroids, especially at high doses, can lead to liver damage, inflammation, and the development of liver tumors or cancer (hepatocellular carcinoma).

3. **Suppression of Immune Function**: Anabolic steroid use may suppress the immune system, making the body less able to detect and eliminate cancerous cells. This can create an environment conducive to tumor growth and metastasis.

4. **Promotion of Tumor Growth**: Anabolic steroids have been shown to stimulate cell growth and proliferation in certain tissues, including muscle, bone, and prostate tissue. While this effect is desirable for muscle growth and performance enhancement, it may also promote the growth of existing tumors or accelerate the progression of pre-existing cancers.

5. **Behavioral Effects**: Anabolic steroid abuse can lead to changes in behavior and mood, including increased aggression and impulsivity. These behavioral changes may increase the risk of engaging in risky behaviors or lifestyle choices that could contribute to cancer risk, such as tobacco use, alcohol abuse, and poor dietary habits.

6. Individuals considering the use of anabolic steroids should be aware of these potential risks and seek guidance from a qualified healthcare professional.

Unraveling the Origins: Exploring 101 Triggers of Cancer

Trigger 23/101 – Aristolochic Acids

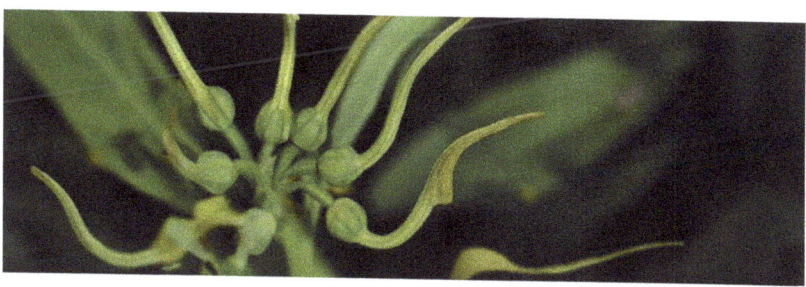

Report: 12th Report on Carcinogens
Carcinogen Category: chemical
Cancer Type(s): kidney

Aristolochic acids are a group of naturally occurring compounds found in plants of the Aristolochia genus and certain plants in the Asarum genus. These compounds are primarily found in the roots, stems, leaves, and seeds of Aristolochia plants and are known for their toxic and carcinogenic properties. Aristolochic acids can form covalent bonds with DNA, creating DNA adducts. These adducts can cause mutations by mispairing during DNA replication, leading to incorrect base incorporation.

Here are some key points about aristolochic acids:

1. **Traditional Use**: Aristolochia plants have been used in traditional medicine systems in various cultures for centuries due to their purported medicinal properties. They have been used to treat a wide range of conditions, including arthritis, gout, snake bites, and digestive disorders.

2. **Toxicity**: Aristolochic acids are highly toxic particularly to the kidneys and urinary tract. Ingestion or exposure to aristolochic acids can cause acute kidney injury, chronic kidney disease,

renal fibrosis, and urinary tract damage.

3. **Carcinogenicity**: Long-term exposure to aristolochic acids has been associated with an increased risk of developing urothelial cancers, including cancers of the urinary bladder, ureter, and renal pelvis. Aristolochic acid-related cancers typically have a characteristic mutation pattern involving the TP53 tumor suppressor gene.

4. **Regulatory Actions**: Due to their toxicity and carcinogenicity, aristolochic acids and products containing them have been banned or restricted in many countries. The International Agency for Research on Cancer (IARC) has classified aristolochic acids as Group 1 carcinogens, indicating that they are known to cause cancer in humans.

5. **Herbal Remedies and Dietary Supplements**: Aristolochia-containing herbal remedies and dietary supplements have been implicated in cases of aristolochic acid poisoning and associated health problems. These products may be marketed for weight loss, detoxification, or other health-related purposes and can pose serious health risks to consumers.

6. **Pharmacological Properties**: Despite their toxicity, aristolochic acids have also been studied for their pharmacological properties, including anti-inflammatory, antimicrobial, and anticancer effects. However, the risks associated with their use generally outweigh any potential benefits.

Due to the serious health risks associated with aristolochic acids, caution should be exercised when using herbal remedies or dietary supplements containing Aristolochia plants or related species. Consumers should avoid products with unclear or unregulated ingredients and consult healthcare professionals if they have concerns about potential exposures or health effects.

Unraveling the Origins: Exploring 101 Triggers of Cancer

Trigger 24/101 – Coal Tar

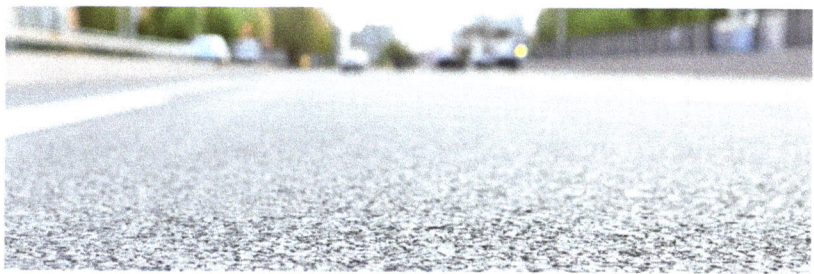

Report: 1st Report on Carcinogens
Carcinogen Category: chemical
Cancer Type(s): lung, scrotal, bladder, kidney

Coal tar is a thick, dark, viscous liquid that is a byproduct of the carbonization of coal during the production of coke or coal gas. It is a complex mixture of organic compounds derived from the distillation of coal at high temperatures in the absence of air. Coal tar contains numerous chemical compounds, including polycyclic aromatic hydrocarbons (PAHs), phenols, and heterocyclic compounds.

Here are some key points about coal tar:

1. **Uses**: Coal tar has historically been used for various industrial and commercial purposes due to its unique properties. It has been used as a sealant and waterproofing agent for roads, roofs, and other structures. It has also been used in the manufacture of asphalt, pitch, creosote, and other industrial chemicals. Additionally, coal tar has been used in traditional medicine for the treatment of skin conditions such as psoriasis, eczema, and dandruff.

2. **Health Effects**: Coal tar and coal tar products are known to contain numerous toxic and carcinogenic compounds,

including PAHs such as benzo[a]pyrene, which is classified as a Group 1 carcinogen by the International Agency for Research on Cancer (IARC). Prolonged or excessive exposure to coal tar can increase the risk of skin cancer, particularly in workers involved in coal tar processing or in industries that use coal tar-derived products.

3. **Environmental Impact**: Coal tar and coal tar-derived products can pose environmental risks due to their potential to leach toxic compounds into soil, water, and air. Contamination of soil and groundwater with PAHs from coal tar can pose risks to human health and ecosystems. Efforts to mitigate environmental contamination from coal tar often involve remediation and cleanup efforts, as well as regulations on the use and disposal of coal tar products.

Overall, while coal tar has historically been valued for its industrial and medicinal properties, its toxic and carcinogenic nature has led to concerns about its safety and environmental impact.

Trigger 25/101 – Secondhand Tobacco Smoke

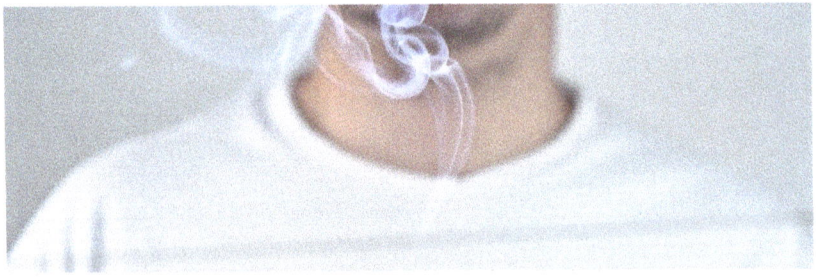

Report: 9th Report on Carcinogens
Carcinogen Category: chemical
Cancer Type(s): lung, bladder, breast

Unraveling the Origins: Exploring 101 Triggers of Cancer

Secondhand tobacco smoke, also known as passive smoke or environmental tobacco smoke (ETS), is classified as a Group 1 carcinogen by the International Agency for Research on Cancer (IARC). Here are several reasons why secondhand tobacco smoke is considered a carcinogen:

1. **Chemical Composition**: Secondhand smoke is a complex mixture of over 7,000 chemicals, including at least 250 known to be harmful and more than 70 that are known carcinogens. These carcinogens include benzene, formaldehyde, polycyclic aromatic hydrocarbons (PAHs), and N-nitrosamines, among others.

2. **Exposure to Toxic and Carcinogenic Compounds**: When non-smokers are exposed to secondhand smoke, they inhale many of the same toxic and carcinogenic compounds found in tobacco smoke. These compounds can penetrate deep into the lungs and enter the bloodstream, increasing the risk of cancer and other health problems.

3. **Increased Cancer Risk**: Secondhand smoke has been linked to an increased risk of several types of cancer, including lung cancer, nasal sinus cancer, pharyngeal cancer, laryngeal cancer, bladder cancer, and breast cancer. Non-smokers exposed to secondhand smoke, particularly in indoor environments such as homes, workplaces, and public spaces, are at higher risk of developing these cancers compared to non-exposed individuals.

4. **Synergistic Effects**: Secondhand smoke exposure may interact with other environmental and lifestyle factors to further increase the risk of cancer. For example, non-smokers who are exposed to secondhand smoke and also have other risk factors such as genetic predisposition or occupational exposures to

carcinogens may be at even higher risk of developing cancer.

5. **Vulnerable Populations**: Certain populations may be particularly vulnerable to the carcinogenic effects of secondhand smoke, including children, pregnant women, elderly individuals, and individuals with pre-existing health conditions. Children exposed to secondhand smoke are at increased risk of developing respiratory infections, asthma, sudden infant death syndrome (SIDS), and other health problems.

6. **Cumulative Exposure**: The carcinogenic effects of secondhand smoke can accumulate over time with repeated or prolonged exposure. Even brief exposure to secondhand smoke can cause immediate harm to the body, and long-term exposure can significantly increase the risk of cancer and other chronic diseases.

Overall, secondhand tobacco smoke is a significant public health concern due to its well-established carcinogenic properties and its association with a wide range of adverse health effects. Efforts to reduce exposure to secondhand smoke, such as implementing smoke-free policies in public places and promoting smoke-free environments in homes and workplaces, are important for protecting public health and reducing the burden of tobacco-related diseases.

Unraveling the Origins: Exploring 101 Triggers of Cancer

Trigger 26/101 – Tamoxifen

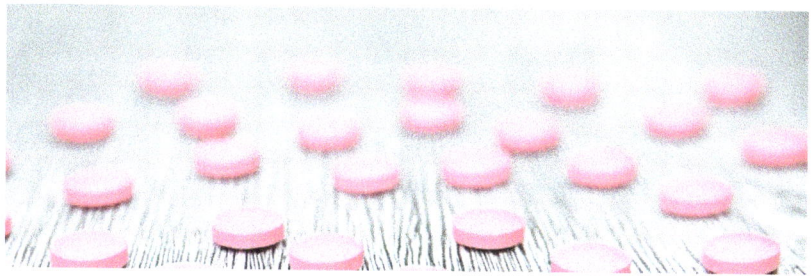

Report: 9th Report on Carcinogens
Carcinogen Category: chemical
Cancer Type(s): uterus

Tamoxifen is a medication that belongs to a class of drugs known as selective estrogen receptor modulators (SERMs). It is commonly used in the treatment and prevention of certain types of breast cancer, particularly hormone receptor-positive breast cancer.

Tamoxifen works by selectively binding to estrogen receptors in breast tissue, thereby blocking the effects of estrogen. Estrogen is a hormone that can promote the growth of some types of breast cancer cells. By blocking estrogen receptors, tamoxifen inhibits the growth and proliferation of hormone-sensitive breast cancer cells.

Tamoxifen may be used to reduce the risk of developing breast cancer in women at high risk of the disease, such as those with a strong family history of breast cancer or certain genetic mutations (e.g., BRCA1 or BRCA2 mutations).

Long-term use of tamoxifen has been associated with an increased risk of developing endometrial cancer, which is cancer of the lining of the uterus. This increased risk is thought to be due to the estrogen-like effects of tamoxifen on the uterus.

Below are some key points about the association between tamoxifen and endometrial cancer:

1. **Estrogen-like Effects**: While tamoxifen acts as an anti-estrogen in breast tissue, it can have estrogen-like effects on the lining of the uterus (endometrium). Tamoxifen can stimulate the growth of the endometrial lining, leading to hyperplasia (excessive growth) and, in some cases, the development of endometrial cancer.

2. **Duration of Use**: The risk of endometrial cancer with tamoxifen use appears to be associated with the duration of treatment. Studies have shown that the risk increases with longer durations of tamoxifen therapy, particularly beyond 5 years of use.

3. **Type of Endometrial Cancer**: Endometrial cancer associated with tamoxifen use is often of the type known as endometrial adenocarcinoma. This type of cancer typically arises from the glands in the lining of the uterus and is the most common type of endometrial cancer.

Unraveling the Origins: Exploring 101 Triggers of Cancer

Trigger 27/101 – 4-Aminobiphenyl

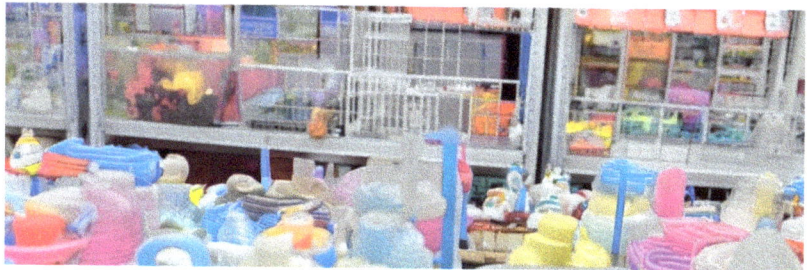

Report: 1st Report on Carcinogens
Carcinogen Category: chemical
Cancer Type(s): bladder

Historically, 4-aminobiphenyl has been used in the production of dyes, pigments, and rubber chemicals. It has also been used in the synthesis of pharmaceuticals and as a research tool in organic chemistry. Exposure to 4-aminobiphenyl has been linked to an increased risk of developing bladder cancer. The carcinogenicity of 4-aminobiphenyl is primarily attributed to its metabolism in the body, where it is converted into reactive intermediates that can damage DNA and lead to the formation of cancerous cells.

4-aminobiphenyl has been used in the following:

1. **Rubber Chemicals**: 4-Aminobiphenyl has been used in the production of certain rubber chemicals, such as antioxidants and vulcanization accelerators. These chemicals are used in the manufacturing of rubber products, including tires, hoses, and seals.

2. **Dyes and Pigments**: 4-Aminobiphenyl has been used in the synthesis of azo dyes and pigments, particularly in the textile industry. These dyes were commonly used to color fabrics and other materials.

3. **Pharmaceuticals**: 4-Aminobiphenyl has been used in the synthesis of certain pharmaceutical compounds, particularly in research and development. However, its use in pharmaceuticals is limited due to its carcinogenic properties.

4. **Research and Laboratory Reagents**: 4-Aminobiphenyl may be used as a research tool in organic chemistry laboratories for the synthesis of other compounds or as a reference standard for analytical purposes.

4-Aminobiphenyl is classified as a carcinogen due to its ability to cause cancer in humans. Several factors contribute to its carcinogenicity:

1. **Metabolism**: Upon entering the body, 4-aminobiphenyl undergoes metabolic activation, primarily in the liver. It is metabolized by enzymes in the body to form reactive intermediates, including N-hydroxy-4-aminobiphenyl and N-acetoxy-4-aminobiphenyl. These reactive intermediates can bind to DNA and form DNA adducts, leading to mutations and genetic damage that can initiate cancer development.

2. **DNA Damage**: The reactive intermediates formed during the metabolism of 4-aminobiphenyl can bind to DNA, causing structural changes and DNA damage. This can result in mutations in critical genes involved in cell growth, proliferation, and DNA repair, ultimately leading to the transformation of normal cells into cancerous cells.

3. **Cancer Sites**: 4-Aminobiphenyl is primarily associated with the development of bladder cancer. It is metabolized in the liver and excreted in the urine, where it can come into contact with the lining of the bladder. The reactive intermediates formed from 4-aminobiphenyl metabolism can directly damage the bladder tissue, leading to the formation of cancerous tumors.

4. **Animal Studies**: Carcinogenicity studies in laboratory animals, particularly rodents, have demonstrated that exposure to 4-aminobiphenyl is associated with an increased incidence of bladder cancer. These animal studies provide evidence of the carcinogenic potential of 4-aminobiphenyl and support its classification as a human carcinogen.

Overall, the carcinogenicity of 4-aminobiphenyl is primarily attributed to its metabolism in the body, which leads to the formation of reactive intermediates that can damage DNA and initiate cancer development, particularly in the bladder. Efforts to minimize exposure to 4-aminobiphenyl and other aromatic amines are important for preventing cancer and protecting human health.

Trigger 28/101 – Estrogen Replacement Therapy

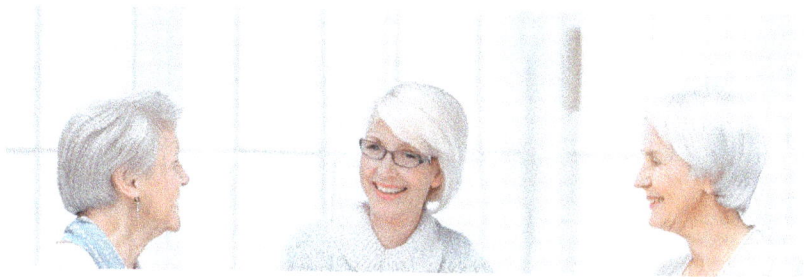

Report: 4th Report on Carcinogens
Carcinogen Category: chemical
Cancer Type(s): breast, ovarian, endometrial.

Estrogen replacement therapy (ERT), also known as hormone replacement therapy (HRT) with estrogen, involves the administration of synthetic or natural estrogen hormones to replace or supplement the estrogen that the body no longer produces in sufficient amounts. Estrogen is a hormone primarily produced by the ovaries in premenopausal women, and it plays a key role in regulating the menstrual cycle, maintaining bone density, and supporting various physiological functions.

Here are some key points about estrogen replacement therapy:

1. **Indications**: Estrogen replacement therapy is primarily used to alleviate symptoms associated with estrogen deficiency, particularly during and after menopause. These symptoms may include hot flashes, night sweats, vaginal dryness, mood swings, and sleep disturbances. ERT can also help prevent or treat certain health conditions associated with estrogen deficiency, such as osteoporosis and vaginal atrophy.

2. **Types of Estrogen**: Estrogen replacement therapy may involve the use of different types of estrogen hormones, including:

   - Estradiol: The most potent and commonly used form of estrogen, which is structurally similar to the estrogen produced by the ovaries.
   - Conjugated estrogens: A mixture of estrogens derived from the urine of pregnant mares, often used in combination with other hormones in hormone replacement therapy.
   - Synthetic estrogens: Estrogen-like compounds that are structurally similar to natural estrogen but are synthesized in a laboratory.

3. **Combination Therapy**: In some cases, estrogen replacement therapy may be combined with progestin (synthetic progesterone) in women who have an intact uterus. This combination helps protect the uterine lining (endometrium) from the potential risk of endometrial hyperplasia or cancer associated with estrogen-alone therapy.

Unraveling the Origins: Exploring 101 Triggers of Cancer

Estrogen replacement therapy is associated with certain risks and side effects, including an increased risk of blood clots, stroke, heart disease, breast cancer, and endometrial cancer (when estrogen is used without progestin in women with an intact uterus). The benefits and risks of estrogen replacement therapy should be carefully weighed and discussed with a healthcare provider before initiating treatment.

Trigger 29/101 – MOOP Chemotherapy

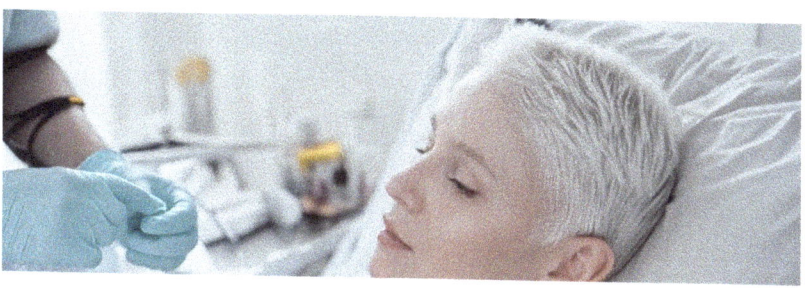

Report: 2nd Report on Carcinogens
Carcinogen Category: chemical
Cancer Type(s): brain, lymphoma, leukemia

MOOP chemotherapy is a chemotherapy regimen used in the treatment of certain types of cancer, particularly Hodgkin lymphoma. The acronym "MOOP" stands for the drugs that are typically included in this regimen:

1. **Mechlorethamine (also known as mustine):** A nitrogen mustard alkylating agent that interferes with the DNA replication process in cancer cells, leading to cell death.

2. **Oncovin (vincristine):** A vinca alkaloid that disrupts microtubule formation, preventing cancer cells from dividing and proliferating.

3. **O**ncovin (procarbazine): An alkylating agent that inhibits DNA and RNA synthesis in cancer cells, leading to cell death.

4. **Prednisone**: A corticosteroid that has anti-inflammatory and immunosuppressive properties, often used in combination with other chemotherapy drugs to enhance their effectiveness and manage side effects such as nausea and vomiting.

It belongs to a class of drugs called alkylating agents, which are known to damage DNA in cells. While this property makes them effective in treating cancer by interfering with the replication and growth of cancer cells, it also poses a risk of causing mutations in healthy cells.

These mutations can lead to the development of secondary cancers, particularly leukemia. Exposure to mechlorethamine has been associated with an increased risk of secondary cancers, including acute myeloid leukemia (AML) and myelodysplastic syndromes (MDS), especially when used in high doses or in combination with other chemotherapy drugs.

Trigger 30/101 – Analgesic Mixtures Containing Phenacetin

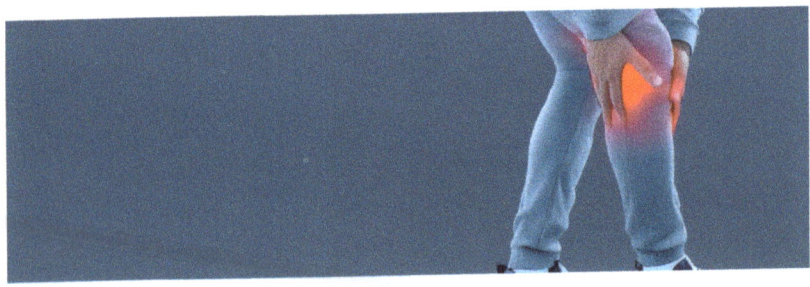

Report: 4th Report on Carcinogens
Carcinogen Category: chemical
Cancer Type(s): liver, kidney, urinary-tract cancer

Unraveling the Origins: Exploring 101 Triggers of Cancer

Analgesic mixtures are combinations of different drugs or substances formulated to relieve pain. These mixtures typically include a variety of compounds that work together to alleviate different types of pain, such as headaches, muscle aches, arthritis pain, menstrual cramps, and so on.

Common ingredients found in analgesic mixtures include:

1. **Nonsteroidal anti-inflammatory drugs (NSAIDs)**: These drugs reduce inflammation and relieve pain. Examples include ibuprofen, aspirin, and naproxen.

2. **Acetaminophen (paracetamol)**: It's a pain reliever and fever reducer, often used in combination with NSAIDs for enhanced pain relief.

3. **Opioids**: These are potent pain relievers that work by binding to opioid receptors in the brain, spinal cord, and other areas of the body. Examples include codeine, morphine, and oxycodone. Opioids are usually reserved for severe pain due to their potential for addiction and side effects.

4. **Muscle relaxants**: These drugs help alleviate muscle spasms and tension, providing relief for conditions such as back pain or muscle strains.

5. **Caffeine**: Sometimes included in analgesic mixtures to enhance the effectiveness of other pain relievers, especially for headaches.

Analgesic mixtures are available in various forms such as tablets, capsules, powders, liquids, and topical creams or gels. They are commonly used for both acute and chronic pain management, but it's essential to use them according to the recommended dosage

and under the guidance of a healthcare professional to minimize the risk of adverse effects and drug interactions.
Top of Form

Phenacetin is a synthetic compound that was formerly used as an analgesic (pain reliever) and antipyretic (fever reducer). It was widely used in over the counter and prescription medications for several decades, primarily in the late 19th and early to mid-20th centuries. Phenacetin was valued for its ability to relieve mild to moderate pain, especially headaches, and it was often combined with other drugs like aspirin and caffeine in analgesic mixtures.

However, due to concerns about its safety, phenacetin has been largely withdrawn from the market in many countries. Research linked phenacetin to kidney damage, particularly when used chronically or in high doses. Additionally, it has been associated with an increased risk of certain cancers, such as renal and bladder cancer.

As a result of these health concerns, regulatory agencies in many countries have banned or severely restricted the use of phenacetin in pharmaceuticals. In the United States, for example, the FDA banned phenacetin in 1983.

While phenacetin itself is no longer widely used, its historical significance lies in its role as one of the first synthetic drugs to gain widespread use as an analgesic. However, due to its adverse effects, it has largely been replaced by safer alternatives such as acetaminophen (paracetamol) and NSAIDs like ibuprofen and aspirin.

Phenacetin has been associated with an increased risk of cancer, particularly kidney and bladder cancer, based on epidemiological studies and animal research. Below are several potential reasons

Unraveling the Origins: Exploring 101 Triggers of Cancer

why it's a carcinogen:

1. **Metabolism**: Phenacetin is metabolized in the body to produce various compounds, some of which may be carcinogenic or toxic to cells. One of its metabolites, called p-phenetidine, can be converted into substances that damage DNA, potentially leading to cancerous changes in cells.

2. **Oxidative stress**: Phenacetin metabolism can generate reactive oxygen species (ROS), which are molecules known to cause oxidative stress and damage to cellular components, including DNA. Prolonged exposure to oxidative stress can increase the risk of cancer development.

3. **Renal toxicity**: Phenacetin has been shown to cause kidney damage, including renal papillary necrosis, a condition characterized by cell death in the renal papilla. Chronic kidney damage and inflammation may promote the development of kidney cancer over time.

4. **Bladder irritation**: Phenacetin and its metabolites can be excreted in urine, potentially exposing the bladder lining to carcinogenic compounds. Chronic irritation and inflammation of the bladder epithelium may increase the likelihood of bladder cancer development.

Pain is mostly associated with inflammation. There are numerous alternatives to reduce inflammation naturally.

Trigger 31/101 – Arsenic

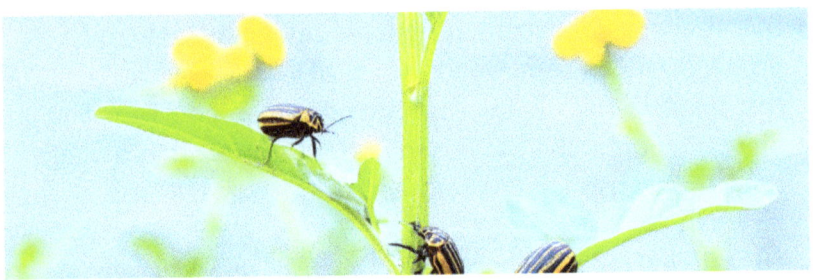

Report: 1st Report on Carcinogens
Carcinogen Category: environment
Cancer Type(s): stomach, lung, leukemia, lymphoma

Arsenic is a naturally occurring chemical element with the symbol As and atomic number 33. It belongs to the group of metalloids, which are elements that have properties intermediate between metals and nonmetals.

Arsenic is widely distributed in the Earth's crust and can be found in various minerals and ores. It exists in several different forms, including inorganic arsenic compounds and organic arsenic compounds. Inorganic arsenic compounds are generally considered more toxic than organic forms.

Historically, arsenic has been used for various purposes due to its toxicity and chemical properties. Some common uses of arsenic have included:

1. **Pesticides**: Arsenic-based compounds were once widely used as insecticides, herbicides, and fungicides in agriculture. However, many of these uses have been phased out or banned due to environmental and health concerns.

2. **Medicine**: In the past, arsenic compounds were used in traditional medicines for the treatment of various ailments,

including syphilis and skin diseases. However, these uses have largely been abandoned due to the toxic effects of arsenic.

3. **Wood preservatives**: Arsenic compounds, such as chromated copper arsenate (CCA), were used to treat wood to prevent decay and insect damage in outdoor applications like decks, fences, and playground equipment. However, CCA-treated wood has been phased out of consumer products due to concerns about arsenic leaching into the environment.

Arsenic is highly toxic to humans and other organisms, primarily affecting the cardiovascular, respiratory, gastrointestinal, and nervous systems. Chronic exposure to low levels of arsenic in drinking water or food can lead to a variety of health problems, including skin lesions, cancer (such as skin, lung, bladder, and liver cancer), cardiovascular disease, and neurological disorders.

Due to its toxicity and potential health risks, arsenic exposure is a significant environmental and public health concern. Efforts to monitor and regulate arsenic levels in drinking water, food, and consumer products are essential for protecting human health and minimizing exposure to this hazardous substance.

Arsenic can be found in various products and substances, both naturally occurring and because of human activities. Here are some common sources of arsenic:

1. **Drinking Water**: Arsenic can contaminate groundwater in certain regions, particularly in areas with natural geological formations that release arsenic into the water. Drinking water from wells in these areas may contain elevated levels of arsenic.

2. **Food**: Arsenic can be present in certain foods, particularly seafood, rice, and some fruits and vegetables. Seafood may contain organic forms of arsenic, while rice and other crops

can accumulate inorganic arsenic from soil and water.

3. **Herbicides and Pesticides**: Arsenic-based compounds were once widely used as herbicides, insecticides, and fungicides in agriculture. While many of these uses have been phased out or banned, traces of arsenic may still be present in soil and water in agricultural areas.

4. **Wood Preservatives**: Arsenic compounds, such as chromated copper arsenate (CCA), were used to treat wood to prevent decay and insect damage. CCA-treated wood was commonly used for outdoor structures like decks, fences, and playground equipment. Although its use has been phased out in consumer products, older structures may still contain CCA-treated wood.

5. **Consumer Products**: Arsenic may be present in certain consumer products, such as cosmetics, particularly those containing rice-based ingredients or certain minerals. Arsenic contamination has also been found in some herbal supplements and traditional medicines.

6. **Industrial Processes**: Arsenic may be released into the environment as a byproduct of certain industrial processes, such as mining, smelting, and coal burning. Industrial activities can contribute to arsenic contamination of air, water, and soil in surrounding areas.

7. **Soil and Dust**: Arsenic can naturally occur in soil and may be present in dust particles in indoor and outdoor environments. People may be exposed to arsenic by ingesting contaminated soil or inhaling airborne particles.

While the use of inorganic arsenic in the United States has been significantly reduced and is tightly regulated, it has not been eliminated. Specific industrial applications and legacy uses persist,

Unraveling the Origins: Exploring 101 Triggers of Cancer

but they are subject to stringent regulatory controls aimed at protecting human health and the environment.

Trigger 32/101 – Auramine

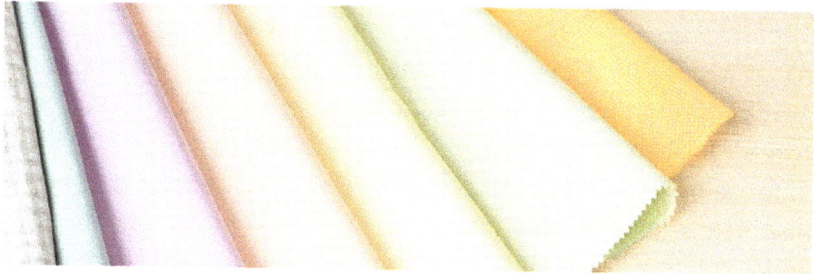

Report: 12th Report on Carcinogens
Carcinogen Category: chemical
Cancer Type(s): bladder

Auramine is a synthetic dye that belongs to the family of diarylmethane dyes. It is commonly used as a fluorescent stain in microbiology and histology for the detection of acid-fast bacteria, particularly Mycobacterium species such as Mycobacterium tuberculosis, the causative agent of tuberculosis.

When used as a stain, auramine binds to the lipid-rich cell walls of acid-fast bacteria and fluoresces under specific wavelengths of light, allowing for their visualization under a fluorescence microscope. This staining technique is known as the auramine-rhodamine stain or the auramine O method.

The auramine-rhodamine staining technique is widely used in clinical laboratories for the rapid detection of acid-fast bacilli in clinical specimens, such as sputum, bronchial washings, and tissue biopsies. It is a crucial diagnostic tool for the early detection and diagnosis of tuberculosis, allowing healthcare providers to initiate appropriate treatment and infection control measures promptly.

In addition to its use in microbiology, auramine has also found applications in other fields, including textile dyeing, ink production, and fluorescence microscopy for the visualization of various biological structures and molecules.

The potential carcinogenicity of auramine arises from its chemical structure and properties. Like many aromatic amines and dyes, auramine can undergo metabolic activation in the body, leading to the formation of reactive intermediates that can bind to DNA and proteins, potentially causing mutations and cellular damage. These reactive metabolites may also interfere with cellular processes involved in DNA repair and cell cycle regulation, further contributing to carcinogenesis.

In experimental studies, auramine has been shown to induce tumors in laboratory animals, particularly when administered at high doses or for prolonged periods. However, the relevance of these findings to human health is uncertain, and additional research is needed to fully understand the potential risks associated with exposure to auramine in humans.

It's important to note that the carcinogenicity of auramine primarily applies to occupational settings where workers may be exposed to high levels of the dye, such as in dye manufacturing facilities or laboratories. Proper safety measures, including ventilation, personal protective equipment, and adherence to recommended exposure limits, can help minimize the risk of exposure to auramine and other potentially carcinogenic substances in the workplace.

Unraveling the Origins: Exploring 101 Triggers of Cancer

Trigger 33/101 – Benzo[a]pyrene

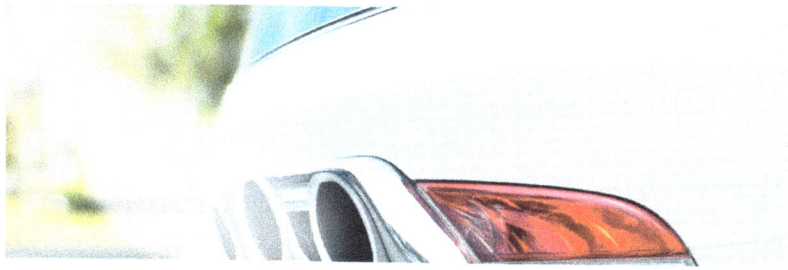

Report: 2nd Report on Carcinogens
Carcinogen Category: chemical
Cancer Type(s): lung, stomach, skin, bladder

Benzo[a]pyrene is primarily formed during the incomplete combustion of organic matter, such as tobacco smoke, vehicle exhaust, industrial emissions, and the burning of fossil fuels and biomass. It is also produced during the cooking of certain foods at high temperatures, such as grilling, frying, or smoking meats.

Exposure to benzo[a]pyrene occurs through inhalation of contaminated air, consumption of contaminated food and water, and dermal contact with contaminated soil or surfaces. Once absorbed into the body, benzo[a]pyrene can undergo metabolic activation by enzymes in the liver, resulting in the formation of reactive intermediates that can bind to DNA and form DNA adducts. These DNA adducts can disrupt normal cellular functions, interfere with DNA repair mechanisms, and ultimately lead to mutations and carcinogenesis.

The carcinogenicity of benzo[a]pyrene has been extensively studied in both laboratory animals and humans. It has been shown to cause a wide range of cancers, including lung cancer, skin cancer, bladder cancer, and gastrointestinal cancers, among others. The International Agency for Research on Cancer (IARC) has classified benzo[a]pyrene as a Group 1 carcinogen, indicating that it is carcinogenic to humans based on sufficient evidence from both experimental studies and epidemiological research.

Several mechanisms contribute to the formation of benzo[a]pyrene during the cooking of meats:

1. **Pyrolysis:** When meat is cooked at high temperatures, organic compounds present in the meat, such as fats and proteins, undergo pyrolysis, which is the chemical decomposition or breakdown of organic molecules due to heat. Pyrolysis of these compounds can lead to the formation of polycyclic aromatic hydrocarbons (PAHs), including benzo[a]pyrene.

2. **Fat dripping and flare-ups:** When fat drips onto hot surfaces, such as grill grates or charcoal, it can cause flare-ups and the production of smoke. The smoke contains PAHs, including benzo[a]pyrene, which can adhere to the surface of the meat and contribute to its contamination.

3. **Incomplete combustion:** Incomplete combustion of organic matter, such as wood, charcoal, or propane, used for grilling or smoking meats, can lead to the formation of PAHs, including benzo[a]pyrene, in the smoke that comes into contact with the meat.

4. **Direct contact with flames or charred surfaces:** When meats are grilled or barbecued directly over an open flame or on charred surfaces, they may come into direct contact with PAHs formed from the combustion of organic matter, leading to the deposition of these compounds on the surface of the meat.

Unraveling the Origins: Exploring 101 Triggers of Cancer

Trigger 34/101 – Beryllium

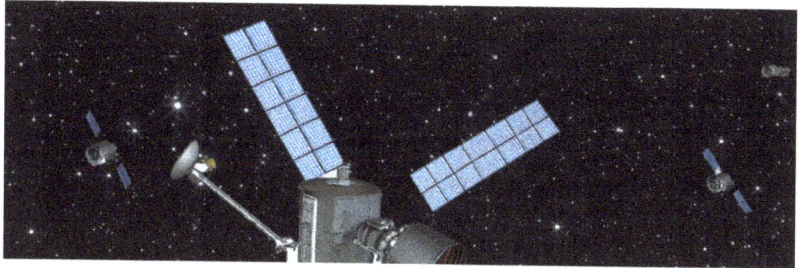

Report: 2nd Report on Carcinogens
Carcinogen Category: chemical
Cancer Type(s): lung

Beryllium is a lightweight, silver-gray metal that is relatively rare in the Earth's crust. Beryllium has a high melting point, excellent thermal conductivity, and is non-magnetic and non-sparking. These properties make it valuable for various industrial applications.

Chronic beryllium disease (CBD) is an inflammatory lung condition that occurs in individuals who have been exposed to beryllium dust or fumes over an extended period, usually through occupational exposure in industries such as aerospace, electronics, and metalworking. In CBD, the body's immune system reacts to beryllium particles, leading to the formation of granulomas (small nodules of immune cells) in the lungs. Over time, these granulomas can cause scarring and fibrosis of lung tissue, leading to symptoms such as shortness of breath, coughing, and fatigue.

Beryllium and its compounds have various industrial applications. Beryllium is used in aerospace components, such as satellite structures, mirrors for telescopes and missile guidance systems, and thermal protection systems for spacecraft.

Studies have suggested that individuals with CBD may have an increased risk of developing lung cancer compared to the general population. The exact mechanism by which CBD predisposes individuals to lung cancer is not fully understood, but it is thought to be related to the chronic inflammation and tissue damage caused by beryllium exposure. Chronic inflammation is a known risk factor for cancer development, as it can lead to DNA damage, genetic mutations, and alterations in cell signaling pathways that regulate cell growth and proliferation.

Beryllium is used in the production of electrical contacts, connectors, and heat sinks for electronic devices, where its high thermal conductivity and low coefficient of thermal expansion are beneficial.

Beryllium alloys are used in X-ray windows, dental alloys, and other medical devices due to their strength, light weight, and biocompatibility.

Despite its valuable properties, beryllium is also toxic, particularly in the form of beryllium dust or fumes, which can cause chronic beryllium disease (CBD), a serious lung condition. Therefore, proper safety measures must be taken when handling beryllium and its compounds to prevent exposure and minimize health risks.

Unraveling the Origins: Exploring 101 Triggers of Cancer

Trigger 35/101 – Betel Quid

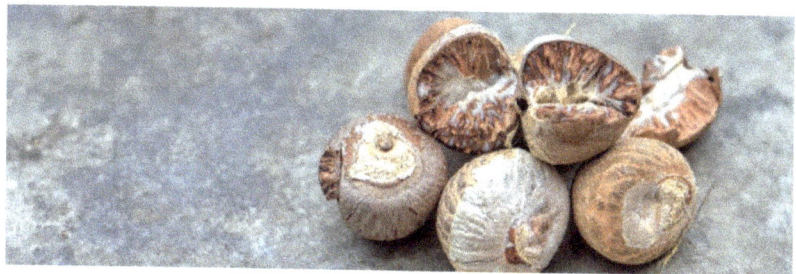

Report: IARC 2003
Carcinogen Category: chemical
Cancer Type(s): oral, pharynx, and oesophagus

Betel quid, also known simply as betel, is a mixture of ingredients commonly chewed for their stimulant and psychoactive effects in many parts of Asia and the Pacific. It is prepared by wrapping betel leaf around areca nut (the seed of the Areca catechu palm), often with slaked lime (calcium hydroxide) and sometimes mixed with tobacco. Sometimes, other ingredients like spices, sweeteners, or condiments may also be added.

The components of betel quid have various effects:

1. **Areca Nut**: Contains alkaloids such as arecoline, which acts as a central nervous system stimulant and can produce feelings of euphoria and increased alertness. However, it is also associated with various health risks, including addiction, cardiovascular effects, and an increased risk of oral cancer.

2. **Betel Leaf**: The leaf of the Piper betle plant, which contains aromatic compounds and is believed to have mild stimulant and digestive properties.

3. **Slaked Lime**: Also known as calcium hydroxide, it is used to enhance the alkalinity of the mixture and facilitate the release of arecoline from the areca nut. It is also thought to have antimicrobial properties and aid in digestion.

4. **Tobacco (optional)**: Some preparations of betel quid include tobacco, which adds nicotine to the mixture and enhances its stimulant effects. However, this also increases the health risks associated with betel quid, including addiction and an increased risk of oral cancer and other health problems associated with tobacco use.

Betel quid chewing is deeply ingrained in many cultures and is often associated with social and ceremonial events. It is commonly used as a mild stimulant, to freshen breath, aid in digestion, and as a traditional remedy for various ailments. However, long-term use of betel quid, especially when combined with tobacco, is associated with a range of health risks, including oral cancer, gum disease, cardiovascular disease, and addiction. Therefore, health authorities in many countries advise against the use of betel quid, particularly in combination with tobacco.

Unraveling the Origins: Exploring 101 Triggers of Cancer

Trigger 36/101 – Bis(chloromethyl)ether and Chloromethyl Methyl Ether

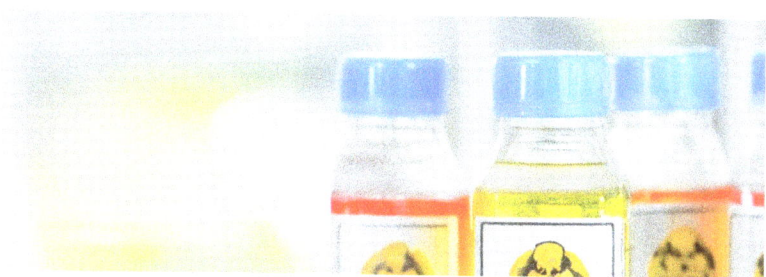

Report: 1ˢᵗ Report on Carcinogens
Carcinogen Category: chemical
Cancer Type(s): lung

Bis(chloromethyl)ether, often abbreviated as BCME, is a highly toxic chemical. It was used in industry as a chemical intermediate in the production of plastics, resins, rubber to increase adhesion, flame-retardant fabrics and dyes, as well as a cross-linking agent in the manufacture of certain polymers.
However, BCME is extremely hazardous to human health and has been classified as a potent carcinogen by several health and regulatory agencies, including the International Agency for Research on Cancer (IARC). Inhalation or skin exposure to BCME can cause severe damage to the respiratory system and skin, as well as an increased risk of developing cancers such as lung cancer and mesothelioma.

Due to its extreme toxicity and carcinogenicity, the use of BCME has been heavily restricted or banned in many countries, and safer alternatives have been developed for the industrial processes where BCME was once used. Strict safety regulations and guidelines are in place for handling and disposing of BCME and contaminated materials to minimize the risk of exposure and protect human health and the environment.

CMME has been used in industrial processes as a reagent for the synthesis of other chemicals, including pharmaceuticals, pesticides, and plastics. It has also been used as a solvent and as a component in the manufacture of certain polymers.

Workers in industries that produced or use BCME or its precursors (such as certain chemical manufacturing processes) are at risk. In areas with older industrial sites where BCME was used or produced, there may be residual contamination.

Trigger 37/101 – 1,3-Butadiene

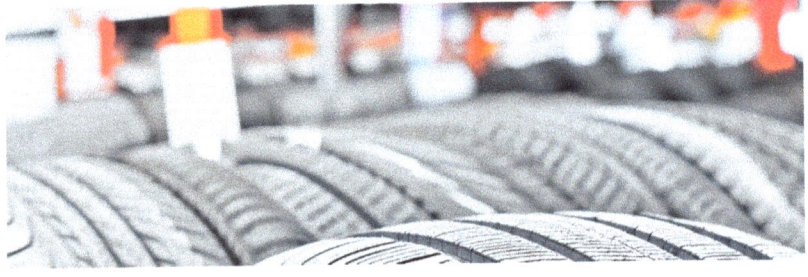

Report: 1st Report on Carcinogens
Carcinogen Category: chemical
Cancer Type(s): lung

Butadiene is primarily produced as a byproduct of the steam cracking of hydrocarbons, particularly ethylene, during the refining of crude oil or the production of other petrochemicals. It is widely used in the production of synthetic rubbers, specifically styrene-butadiene rubber (SBR) and polybutadiene rubber (BR), which are important materials in the manufacture of tires, hoses, belts, gaskets, and various other rubber products.

Apart from its role in rubber production, butadiene is also used as a chemical intermediate in the synthesis of various other compounds, including plastics, resins, coatings, adhesives, and synthetic fibers. It is also used as a monomer in the production of certain types of synthetic elastomers and thermoplastics.

While butadiene is an important industrial chemical, it is also considered hazardous to human health and the environment. Inhalation or skin exposure to butadiene can cause irritation to the respiratory system and skin. Moreover, long-term exposure to butadiene has been associated with an increased risk of certain cancers, particularly leukemia and lymphoma. Therefore, strict safety regulations and guidelines are in place for the handling, storage, and disposal of butadiene and products containing it to minimize the risk of exposure and protect human health and the environment.

Butadiene is classified as a known human carcinogen by several health and regulatory agencies, including the International Agency for Research on Cancer (IARC), the United States Environmental Protection Agency (EPA), and the National Toxicology Program (NTP). The carcinogenicity of butadiene is primarily associated with its metabolic activation in the body to reactive intermediates that can interact with cellular DNA, leading to genetic mutations and the development of cancer.

Overall, while the precise mechanisms underlying butadiene-induced carcinogenesis are complex and not fully understood, it is clear that metabolic activation and the formation of reactive intermediates that can damage DNA play a central role in the carcinogenicity of this chemical. Strict occupational and environmental regulations are in place to minimize exposure to butadiene and protect workers and the general population from the associated health risks.

Trigger 38/101 – Captafol

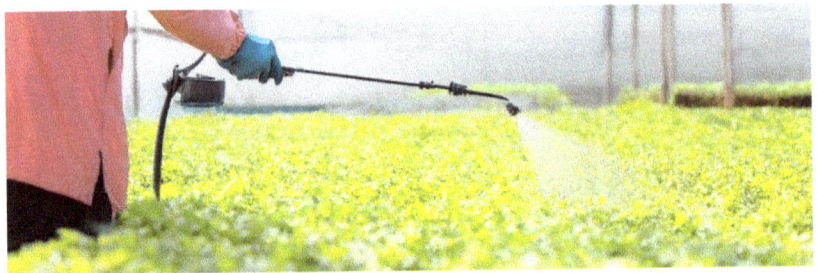

Report: 12th Report on Carcinogens
Carcinogen Category: chemical
Cancer Type(s): lymphoid, blood-vessel, spleen, liver, thyroid

Captafol is a synthetic fungicide that belongs to the organochlorine chemical class. It has been used primarily to control fungal diseases in crops such as fruits, vegetables, nuts, ornamentals, and field crops. Captafol works by inhibiting the growth of fungi, preventing the development of fungal diseases, and protecting crops from damage.

However, due to concerns about its potential toxicity and environmental impact, the use of captafol has been heavily restricted or banned in many countries. Captafol has been classified as a possible human carcinogen by the International Agency for Research on Cancer (IARC), based on animal studies showing an increased incidence of tumors, particularly liver and thyroid tumors, in rats and mice exposed to captafol. Additionally, captafol has been associated with reproductive and developmental toxicity in animal studies, as well as adverse effects on the endocrine system. Concerns about its persistence in the environment and potential for bioaccumulation have also contributed to regulatory restrictions on its use.

Unraveling the Origins: Exploring 101 Triggers of Cancer

As a result, many countries have phased out or banned the use of captafol, and safer alternatives have been developed for the control of fungal diseases in agriculture. Strict regulations are in place for the handling, storage, and disposal of captafol and products containing it to minimize human exposure and environmental contamination.

The reactive metabolites of captafol can form covalent adducts with DNA, leading to DNA damage and genetic mutations. These DNA adducts can disrupt normal DNA replication and repair processes, potentially leading to the development of tumors.

Captafol and its metabolites can induce oxidative stress in cells by generating reactive oxygen species (ROS) and other free radicals. Oxidative stress can cause damage to cellular components, including DNA, proteins, and lipids, and contribute to carcinogenesis.

Trigger 39/101 – Chlorambucil

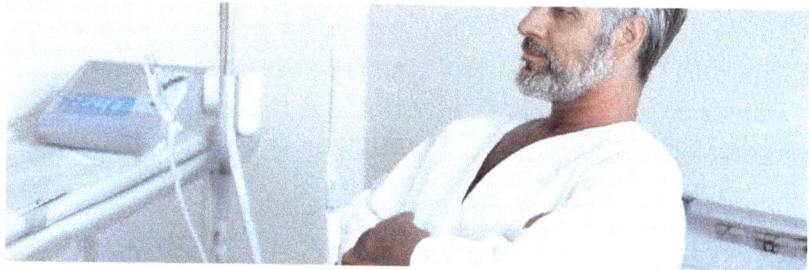

Report: 2nd Report on Carcinogens
Carcinogen Category: chemical
Cancer Type(s): hematopoietic, lymphosarcoma, leukemia

Chlorambucil is a chemotherapy medication that belongs to the class of alkylating agents. It is used primarily in the treatment of various types of cancer, including chronic lymphocytic leukemia (CLL), Hodgkin's disease, non-Hodgkin's lymphoma, and certain types of ovarian cancer.

Chlorambucil works by interfering with the DNA of cancer cells, preventing their replication and ultimately leading to their destruction. It does this by attaching alkyl groups to the DNA molecules, which disrupts their structure and function. This leads to cell death and slows down the growth and spread of cancerous cells.

Chlorambucil carries potential side effects, including:

1. **Bone marrow suppression**: Chlorambucil can reduce the production of blood cells in the bone marrow, leading to anemia, thrombocytopenia (low platelet count), and neutropenia (low white blood cell count). This can increase the risk of infections, bleeding, and fatigue.

2. **Increased risk of infections**: Due to its effects on the bone marrow, chlorambucil can weaken the immune system, increasing the risk of infections.

3. **Long-term side effects**: Prolonged use of chlorambucil may be associated with an increased risk of secondary cancers, such as myelodysplastic syndrome (MDS) or acute myeloid leukemia (AML).

Chlorambucil, while primarily used as a chemotherapy medication to treat cancer, is also classified as a carcinogen itself. The carcinogenicity of chlorambucil is primarily attributed to its mechanism of action and its ability to damage DNA.

Unraveling the Origins: Exploring 101 Triggers of Cancer

Trigger 40/101 – Chlorinated paraffins

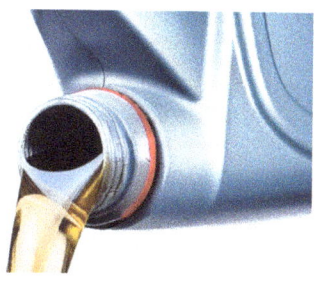

Report: 5th Report on Carcinogens
Carcinogen Category: chemical
Cancer Type(s): liver, thyroid, liver, leukemia

Chlorinated paraffins (CPs) are a group of synthetic chemicals that consist of long-chain hydrocarbons with chlorine atoms attached. They are typically produced by chlorination of straight-chain paraffin hydrocarbons, which are derived from petroleum or other sources.

Chlorinated paraffins are widely used as additives in a variety of industrial and consumer products due to their properties, including:

1. **Flame Retardancy**: Chlorinated paraffins are effective flame retardants and are often added to plastics, rubber, textiles, and other materials to reduce their flammability and improve fire resistance.

2. **Plasticizers**: Chlorinated paraffins can act as plasticizers, which are additives that improve the flexibility, durability, and workability of plastics and other materials. They are commonly used in PVC (polyvinyl chloride) products, such as

vinyl flooring, cables, and synthetic leather.

3. **Metalworking Fluids**: Chlorinated paraffins are used as lubricants and extreme pressure additives in metalworking fluids, such as cutting oils and coolants, to improve machining performance and reduce friction and wear on metal surfaces.

4. **Paints and Coatings**: Chlorinated paraffins are added to paints, coatings, and sealants to enhance their water resistance, adhesion, and durability. They can also improve the flow and leveling properties of paints during application.

5. **Adhesives and Sealants**: Chlorinated paraffins are used as additives in adhesives and sealants to improve their bonding strength, water resistance, and resistance to environmental factors such as temperature and humidity.

While chlorinated paraffins offer several desirable properties for various industrial applications, they have also raised concerns due to their potential environmental and health effects. Some chlorinated paraffins are persistent in the environment and have been detected in soil, water, and wildlife. Additionally, certain types of chlorinated paraffins have been classified as persistent organic pollutants (POPs) and are subject to international regulations under agreements such as the Stockholm Convention on Persistent Organic Pollutants.

Chlorinated paraffins (CPs) have been associated with potential carcinogenicity, primarily due to certain types of CPs containing chlorine atoms with varying degrees of chlorination.

Below are some reasons why chlorinated paraffins are considered to have carcinogenic potential:

Unraveling the Origins: Exploring 101 Triggers of Cancer

1. **Chemical Structure**: CPs consist of long-chain hydrocarbons with chlorine atoms attached. Depending on the degree of chlorination and the distribution of chlorine atoms along the carbon chain, CPs can form reactive intermediates that may interact with cellular DNA and proteins.

2. **Metabolic Activation**: Some CPs undergo metabolic activation in the body, primarily in the liver, by cytochrome P450 enzymes. This metabolic process can convert CPs into reactive intermediates that can react with cellular macromolecules, including DNA, proteins, and lipids.

3. **DNA Damage**: The reactive intermediates formed during the metabolism of CPs can covalently bind to DNA, leading to the formation of DNA adducts. These DNA adducts can disrupt normal DNA replication and repair processes, potentially leading to mutations and chromosomal abnormalities, which are hallmarks of carcinogenesis.

4. **Genotoxicity**: CPs have been shown to exhibit genotoxic effects in experimental studies, meaning they have the potential to directly damage DNA and induce mutations. This genotoxic activity is a key factor in the carcinogenicity of CPs.

5. **Animal Studies**: Animal studies have provided evidence of the carcinogenic potential of certain CPs. In particular, long-term exposure to certain CPs has been associated with an increased incidence of tumors, particularly liver tumors, in laboratory animals.

It is clear that metabolic activation and the formation of reactive intermediates that can damage DNA and disrupt cellular processes play a central role in the carcinogenicity of certain types of CPs. Therefore, regulatory agencies such as the International Agency for Research on Cancer (IARC) have classified certain CPs as possible or probable human carcinogens based on available evidence from animal studies and other sources.

Trigger 41/101 – Semustine (MeCCNU)

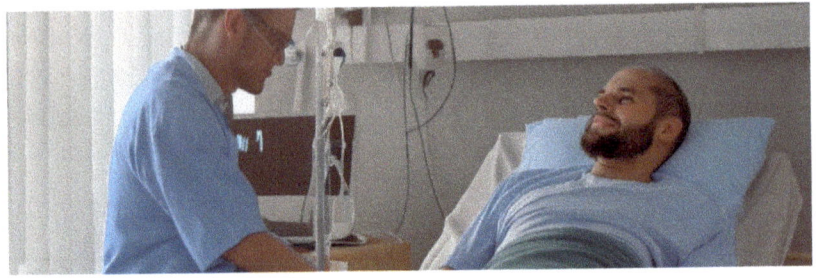

Report: 6th Report on Carcinogens
Carcinogen Category: chemical
Cancer Type(s): leukemia, lung, lymphoma

1-(2-Chloroethyl)-3-(4-methylcyclohexyl)-1-nitrosourea (MeCCNU), also known as semustine, is a chemotherapeutic agent used in the treatment of various types of cancer. It belongs to the class of nitrosourea alkylating agents, which work by interfering with the DNA of cancer cells, preventing their replication and ultimately leading to their destruction.

MeCCNU is primarily used in the treatment of brain tumors, such as glioblastoma multiforme, anaplastic gliomas, and medulloblastoma. It is also used in the treatment of Hodgkin's lymphoma, non-Hodgkin's lymphoma, and certain types of lung cancer.

MeCCNU works by forming reactive compounds that alkylate DNA, leading to the cross-linking of DNA strands and the inhibition of DNA replication and transcription. This ultimately results in cell death and slows down the growth and spread of cancerous cells.

Unraveling the Origins: Exploring 101 Triggers of Cancer

Like other chemotherapy medications, MeCCNU can cause side effects, which may include nausea, vomiting, loss of appetite, fatigue, bone marrow suppression (leading to anemia, thrombocytopenia, and neutropenia), and an increased risk of infections. It may also cause neurological side effects, such as dizziness, confusion, and seizures.

Semustine (1-(2-Chloroethyl)-3-(4-methylcyclohexyl)-1-nitrosourea or MeCCNU) is a member of the nitrosourea class of chemotherapeutic agents. While it is primarily used to treat various types of cancer, including brain tumors and lymphomas, semustine itself is also considered a carcinogen. Here's why:

1. **Alkylating Agent**: Semustine, like other nitrosoureas, works by acting as an alkylating agent. It forms reactive intermediates that can bind to DNA, leading to the formation of DNA adducts. These adducts interfere with DNA replication and transcription, ultimately leading to cell death. However, this process can also lead to mutations in the DNA of both cancerous and healthy cells.

2. **Cross-Linking**: Semustine can cause cross-linking of DNA strands, which can interfere with the normal functioning of the DNA and lead to genetic mutations. These mutations can disrupt normal cellular processes and contribute to the development of cancer.

3. **Genotoxicity**: Semustine has been shown to exhibit genotoxic effects in experimental studies, meaning it has the potential to directly damage DNA and induce mutations. This genotoxic activity is a key factor in the carcinogenicity of semustine.

4. **Secondary Cancers**: Long-term use of semustine as a chemotherapy medication has been associated with an increased risk of developing secondary cancers, particularly

leukemia and other hematological malignancies. This may be due to the genotoxic effects of semustine on bone marrow cells, which can lead to mutations and the development of leukemia.

Semustine carries the risk of causing DNA damage and mutations that can contribute to the development of cancer. Healthcare providers carefully weigh the benefits and risks of semustine treatment when prescribing it to patients, and close monitoring is typically required during and after treatment to minimize the risk of adverse effects, including the development of secondary cancers.

Trigger 42/101 – 2-Chloroethylvinyl Ether

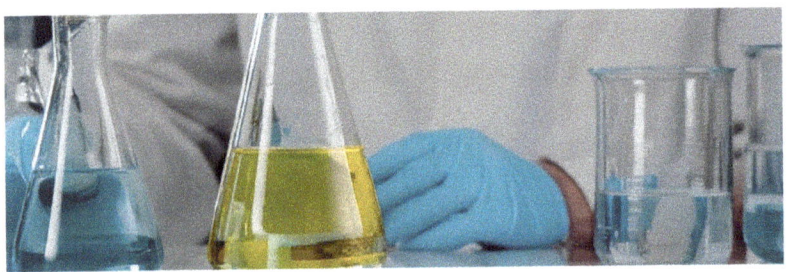

Report: NCIC No. 191
Carcinogen Category: chemical
Cancer Type(s): lung, lymphoma

2-Chloroethylvinyl ether, also known as chloroethyl vinyl ether (CEVE), is primarily used as an intermediate in the synthesis of other organic compounds, including pharmaceuticals, pesticides, and specialty chemicals. CEVE is also used in the production of polymers and copolymers for various industrial applications.

Unraveling the Origins: Exploring 101 Triggers of Cancer

However, CEVE is considered to be toxic and potentially hazardous to human health and the environment. Exposure to CEVE can occur through inhalation, ingestion, or skin contact. It can irritate the respiratory tract, skin, and eyes, and prolonged or repeated exposure may cause more severe health effects, including damage to the liver and kidneys.

Additionally, CEVE has been classified as a possible human carcinogen by the International Agency for Research on Cancer (IARC), based on limited evidence from animal studies suggesting its carcinogenic potential. Therefore, strict safety measures and regulations are in place for the handling, storage, and disposal of CEVE to minimize the risk of exposure and protect human health and the environment.

Chloroethylvinyl ether (CEVE) has been investigated in the past for its potential applications in pharmaceutical chemistry, particularly in the synthesis of certain drugs and pharmaceutical intermediates. For example, it has been used in the synthesis of heterocyclic compounds, which are important structural motifs found in many drugs and pharmaceuticals.

Despite its potential utility as a synthetic building block, the toxic and carcinogenic properties of CEVE pose significant challenges and safety concerns for its use in pharmaceutical applications. As a result, alternative synthetic routes and safer chemical reagents are often preferred in pharmaceutical synthesis to minimize the risk of exposure and ensure the safety of workers and end-users

Eric D Blanks

Trigger 43/101 – Chromium (VI) Compounds

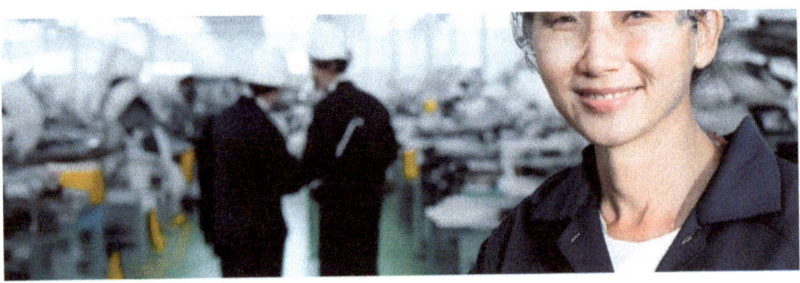

Report: 1st Report on Carcinogens
Carcinogen Category: chemical
Cancer Type(s): lung

Chromium (VI) compounds are used in electroplating processes to provide a hard, corrosion-resistant surface to metals such as steel, aluminum, and zinc. Chromium plating is widely used in the automotive, aerospace, and manufacturing industries.

Chromium (VI) compounds have several other industrial applications, including:

1. **Pigments:** Certain chromium (VI) compounds, such as lead chromate and zinc chromate are used as pigments in paints, coatings, and dyes due to their bright yellow, orange, or green colors.

2. **Wood Preservatives:** Chromium (VI) compounds are used in wood treatment formulations to protect against decay, mold, and insect damage. Chromated copper arsenate (CCA) is a common wood preservative that contains chromium (VI) compounds.

3. **Corrosion Inhibitors:** Some chromium (VI) compounds are used as corrosion inhibitors in cooling water treatment and industrial processes to protect metal surfaces from corrosion.

Unraveling the Origins: Exploring 101 Triggers of Cancer

While chromium (VI) compounds have useful industrial applications, they are also known to pose significant health and environmental risks. Hexavalent chromium is highly toxic and carcinogenic, and exposure to chromium (VI) compounds can lead to adverse health effects, including respiratory problems, skin irritation, allergic reactions, and an increased risk of lung cancer and other cancers.

Due to these health risks, regulatory agencies such as the Environmental Protection Agency (EPA) in the United States have established strict regulations on the use, handling, and disposal of chromium (VI) compounds to protect human health and the environment. Efforts are also underway to develop safer alternatives and technologies to minimize the use and exposure of hexavalent chromium in various industrial processes.

Chromium (VI) compounds are classified as carcinogens due to their ability to cause DNA damage, mutations, and oxidative stress in cells, which can lead to the development of cancer.

Trigger 44/101 – Cobalt Metal with Tungsten Carbide

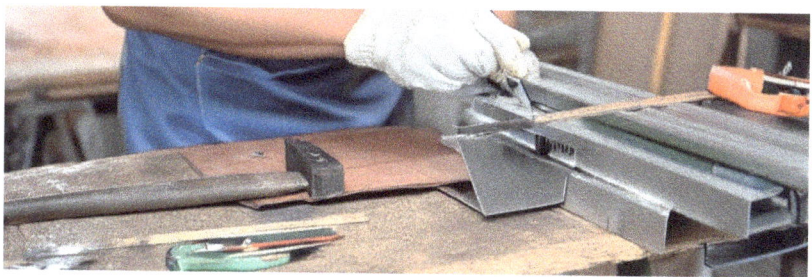

Report: 14th Report on Carcinogens
Category: chemical
Cancer Type(s): leukemia, lung, lymphoma

Cobalt metal with tungsten carbide, often referred to simply as cobalt-tungsten carbide or cobalt-cemented carbide, is a composite material used in various industrial applications, particularly in cutting tools, wear-resistant coatings, and other high-performance applications. It is composed of tungsten carbide particles bonded together by a matrix of cobalt metal.

When cobalt and tungsten carbide are combined, they form a composite material with synergistic properties. The tungsten carbide particles provide exceptional hardness and wear resistance, while the cobalt matrix enhances toughness and impact resistance. This combination makes cobalt-tungsten carbide ideal for applications where extreme hardness, wear resistance, and durability are required, such as cutting, drilling, grinding, and machining operations in metalworking, mining, construction, and other industries.

Common applications of cobalt-tungsten carbide include:

1. Cutting tools (e.g., inserts, drills, end mills, saw blades)

2. Wear-resistant coatings for machinery components

3. Mining and drilling tools

4. Metal forming and shaping tools

5. Surgical instruments and medical devices

6. Aerospace and automotive components

Cobalt metal with tungsten carbide, also known as cemented carbide or hard metal, has been classified as a Group 2B carcinogen (possibly carcinogenic to humans) by the International Agency for Research on Cancer (IARC). Here are some reasons why cobalt metal with tungsten carbide is considered a potential carcinogen:

1. **Cobalt**: Cobalt itself has been classified as a Group 2B carcinogen by the IARC. While the exact mechanisms of cobalt-induced carcinogenesis are not fully understood, animal studies have shown that cobalt compounds can induce tumors at the site of injection or implantation, particularly in the lungs and other tissues. Chronic inhalation or exposure to cobalt dust or fumes has been associated with an increased risk of lung cancer and other respiratory diseases in occupational settings, such as hard metal manufacturing and mining.

2. **Tungsten Carbide**: While tungsten carbide is not inherently carcinogenic, its production and processing can generate fine particulate dust containing cobalt and tungsten carbide particles. Inhalation of these dust particles, especially those containing cobalt, can lead to respiratory tract irritation, inflammation, and fibrosis. Prolonged or chronic exposure to cobalt-containing dust has been linked to an increased risk of lung cancer and other respiratory diseases.

3. **Synergistic Effects**: The carcinogenicity of cobalt metal with tungsten carbide may be enhanced by synergistic effects between cobalt and tungsten carbide particles. Some studies suggest that cobalt may facilitate the cellular uptake and retention of tungsten, potentially increasing its toxic effects and carcinogenic potential in tissues. Additionally, the abrasive nature of tungsten carbide particles may contribute to the deposition of cobalt and other toxicants in the respiratory tract, further increasing the risk of adverse health effects.

4. **Occupational Exposure**: Workers in industries where cobalt metal with tungsten carbide is used or processed, such as hard metal manufacturing, mining, metalworking, and construction, may be at higher risk of exposure to cobalt and tungsten carbide dust. Occupational exposure to cobalt-containing dust has been associated with an increased incidence of lung cancer, asthma, and other respiratory diseases in exposed workers.

Overall, while cobalt metal with tungsten carbide is valued for its hardness, wear resistance, and durability in industrial applications, it is important to minimize occupational exposure to cobalt and tungsten carbide dust to protect workers' health and reduce the risk of carcinogenesis and other adverse health effects associated with exposure to these materials. Adequate ventilation, personal protective equipment (such as respirators), engineering controls, and proper workplace hygiene practices are essential for reducing exposure to cobalt and tungsten carbide dust in occupational settings.

Trigger 45/101 – Combined Estrogen-Progestogen Menopausal Therapy (MHT)

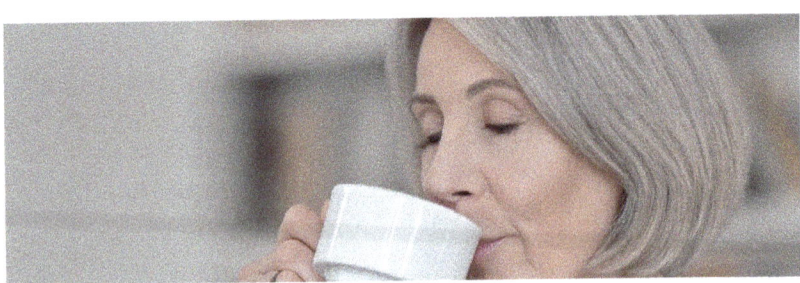

Report: 4th Report on Carcinogens
Category: chemical
Cancer Type(s): breast, ovarian, endometrial

Unraveling the Origins: Exploring 101 Triggers of Cancer

Combined estrogen-progestogen menopausal hormone therapy (MHT), also known as hormone replacement therapy (HRT), is a medical treatment used to relieve symptoms of menopause and prevent or manage certain health conditions associated with menopausal hormonal changes. It involves the administration of both estrogen and progestogen hormones, either separately or in combination, to supplement declining hormone levels in women experiencing menopause.

During menopause, which typically occurs around the age of 45-55, a woman's ovaries gradually produce less estrogen and progesterone hormones, leading to various physical and psychological symptoms. These symptoms may include hot flashes, night sweats, vaginal dryness, mood swings, insomnia, and bone loss (osteoporosis). Additionally, declining estrogen levels increase the risk of certain health conditions, such as osteoporosis, cardiovascular disease, and colorectal cancer.

Combined estrogen-progestogen MHT aims to alleviate menopausal symptoms and reduce the risk of associated health conditions by restoring hormonal balance in the body. Estrogen therapy helps alleviate symptoms such as hot flashes, vaginal dryness, and bone loss by replenishing estrogen levels, while progestogen therapy helps protect the uterine lining (endometrium) from the potential adverse effects of estrogen therapy, such as endometrial hyperplasia and cancer.

The use of hormone therapy is not without risks, and healthcare providers carefully weigh the benefits and potential risks of MHT based on each woman's individual circumstances. Common risks associated with MHT include an increased risk of breast cancer, blood clots, stroke, and cardiovascular disease. Therefore, hormone therapy should be used at the lowest effective dose for the shortest duration necessary to achieve treatment goals.

Regular monitoring and follow-up with a healthcare provider are essential for women receiving combined estrogen-progestogen MHT.

Below are some reasons why MHT is considered to potentially increase cancer risk:

1. **Breast Cancer**: One of the most significant concerns regarding MHT is its association with an increased risk of breast cancer. Studies have shown that long-term use of MHT, particularly estrogen-progestogen combination therapy, is associated with a modestly increased risk of breast cancer. The risk appears to be higher with combination therapy than with estrogen-only therapy, and it may vary depending on factors such as the duration of MHT use, the specific type of hormone therapy, and the individual's underlying risk factors for breast cancer.

2. **Endometrial Cancer**: Estrogen therapy alone (without progestogen) has been associated with an increased risk of endometrial cancer (cancer of the lining of the uterus) because unopposed estrogen can stimulate the growth of the endometrium. However, adding progestogen to estrogen therapy helps protect the endometrium and reduce the risk of endometrial cancer. Therefore, combined estrogen-progestogen therapy is generally preferred over estrogen-only therapy in women with a uterus to mitigate the risk of endometrial cancer.

3. **Ovarian Cancer**: Some studies have suggested that MHT, particularly long-term use of estrogen-progestogen combination therapy, may be associated with a small increased risk of ovarian cancer. However, the evidence for this association is less consistent compared to the associations with breast and endometrial cancers.

Unraveling the Origins: Exploring 101 Triggers of Cancer

It's important to note that the relationship between MHT and cancer risk is complex and influenced by various factors, including the specific type of hormone therapy, the duration and timing of use, the woman's underlying risk factors for cancer, and other lifestyle and environmental factors. Additionally, the overall benefits and risks of MHT should be carefully weighed based on individual circumstances, including the severity of menopausal symptoms, the woman's medical history, and her preferences.

Trigger 46/101 – Contraceptives - Steroidal Estrogens

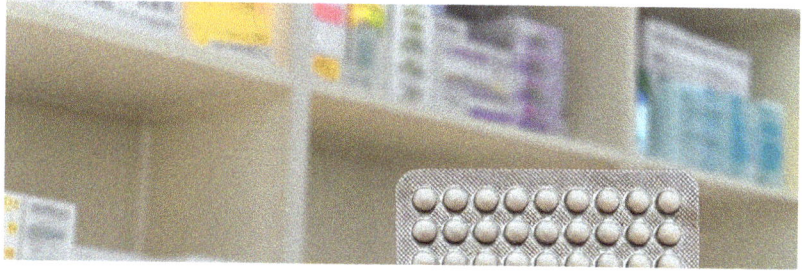

Report: IARC (1999), Volume 72
Category: chemical
Cancer Type(s): endometrial, breast

Contraceptives, also known as birth control or contraception, are methods or devices used to prevent pregnancy by inhibiting the fertilization of an egg by sperm or by preventing implantation of a fertilized egg in the uterus.

Contraceptives play a crucial role in family planning, enabling individuals and couples to make informed decisions about if and when to have children. The choice of contraceptive method depends on factors such as effectiveness, safety, ease of use, personal preferences, and medical considerations. It's essential for individuals to consult with a healthcare provider to determine the most suitable contraceptive option for their needs and circumstances.

Some studies have examined the potential association between the use of certain hormonal contraceptives (specifically, combined estrogen-progestogen contraceptives) and the risk of certain cancers, such as breast and cervical cancer. Below is a breakdown:

1. **Breast Cancer**: Research on the association between hormonal contraceptives and breast cancer risk has yielded mixed findings. Some studies have suggested a slightly increased risk of breast cancer among women who use hormonal contraceptives, particularly those containing high doses of estrogen or progestin. However, the overall risk is considered to be relatively low, especially compared to other risk factors for breast cancer, such as age, family history, and reproductive factors.

2. **Cervical Cancer**: There is some evidence to suggest that long-term use of hormonal contraceptives may be associated with a slightly increased risk of cervical cancer. The risk appears to be higher among women who use hormonal contraceptives for extended periods, particularly those infected with human papillomavirus (HPV), which is a known risk factor for cervical cancer. However, the absolute risk of cervical cancer associated with hormonal contraceptive use is relatively low, and regular cervical cancer screening (e.g., Pap smear) can help detect precancerous changes early and prevent the development of cervical cancer.

It's also worth mentioning that non-hormonal contraceptives, such as barrier methods (e.g., condoms), copper IUDs, and fertility awareness methods, are not associated with an increased risk of cancer and may be suitable alternatives for women who prefer to avoid hormonal contraception or have contraindications to hormonal methods.

Trigger 47/101 – Creosote

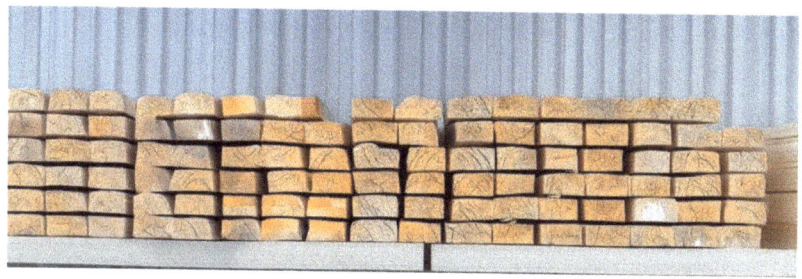

Report: NIH PMID: 10479980
Category: chemical
Cancer Type(s): lung, pancreas, kidney, scrotum, prostate, rectum, bladder

Creosote is a category of chemicals formed by the distillation of tar from wood or coal. It's commonly known for its use as a wood preservative, as it helps protect wood against decay and insects. It's also a concern because it contains several compounds that can be harmful to humans and the environment if not properly handled and disposed of. Exposure to creosote can lead to health issues, so it's important to take precautions when working with or around it.

Creosote is considered a carcinogen because it contains several compounds, such as polycyclic aromatic hydrocarbons (PAHs), that have been linked to cancer in humans. When creosote-treated wood is burned, these compounds can be released into the air and potentially inhaled, increasing the risk of cancer. Additionally, prolonged skin contact with creosote or ingestion of food or water contaminated with creosote residues can also pose a risk of cancer. The International Agency for Research on Cancer (IARC), a specialized cancer agency of the World Health Organization (WHO), has classified creosote as a Group 2A carcinogen, which means it is probably carcinogenic to humans. This classification is based on evidence from studies showing associations between creosote exposure and various types of cancer in humans, as well as evidence from animal studies demonstrating carcinogenic effects.

Creosote is primarily used as a wood preservative in various products and applications. Some common products that may contain creosote-treated wood include:

1. Railroad ties: Creosote is extensively used to treat wooden railroad ties to protect them from decay and insect damage, prolonging their lifespan and ensuring the safety and stability of railroad tracks.

2. Utility poles: Wooden utility poles are often treated with creosote to protect them from rot, insects, and weathering, thereby extending their service life and ensuring reliable electricity transmission and distribution.

3. Marine structures: Creosote-treated wood is used in marine construction for docks, piers, seawalls, and other waterfront structures to resist decay and damage from marine organisms.

4. Outdoor fencing: Wooden fence posts and rails are sometimes treated with creosote to enhance their durability and longevity, particularly in outdoor environments where they are exposed to moisture and pests.

Unraveling the Origins: Exploring 101 Triggers of Cancer

5. Garden and landscaping: Creosote-treated wood may be used for garden edging, retaining walls, and landscaping timbers to provide long-term protection against decay and termites.

6. Playgrounds: Some playground equipment, such as wooden play structures and posts, may be treated with creosote to increase their resistance to decay and insect infestation, although alternative treatments are becoming more common due to health and safety concerns.

It's important to note that while creosote is effective at preserving wood, its use has declined in certain applications due to health and environmental concerns associated with its toxic components. Alternative wood preservatives and treatment methods that are less harmful to human health and the environment are increasingly being used where possible.

Trigger 48/101 – Crystalline Silica

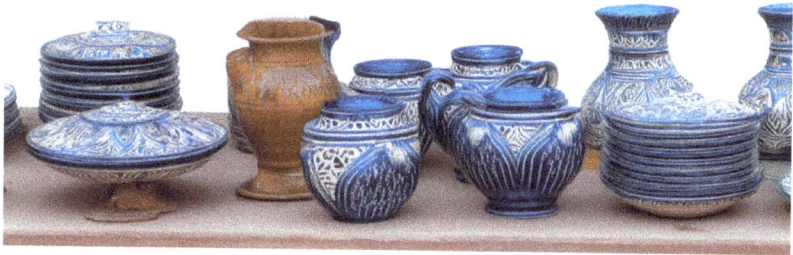

Report: 6th Report on Carcinogens
Category: chemical
Cancer Type(s): lung

Crystalline silica is a naturally occurring mineral found in various types of rocks, such as quartz, sand, and granite. It is commonly used in a wide range of industrial processes and products due to its hardness, stability, and heat resistance. Crystalline silica exists in different forms, including quartz, cristobalite, and tridymite.

In industrial settings, crystalline silica can become airborne during activities such as mining, quarrying, drilling, cutting, grinding, and blasting of materials containing silica. Inhalation of crystalline silica dust can pose serious health risks, particularly to the respiratory system. Prolonged exposure to high levels of crystalline silica dust can lead to lung diseases such as silicosis, lung cancer, and other respiratory problems.

Due to its health hazards, regulatory agencies and occupational health organizations have established exposure limits and guidelines to protect workers from excessive exposure to crystalline silica dust. Employers in industries where crystalline silica is present are required to implement measures to control dust levels, provide personal protective equipment (such as respirators), and offer training on safe handling practices to minimize the risk of exposure.

Silica, in various forms, is widely used in numerous products across different industries due to its versatile properties. Here are some common products that may contain silica:

1. **Construction materials:** Silica sand is a key component in the production of concrete, mortar, and other construction materials due to its high strength and stability. It's also used as a component in various types of bricks, tiles, and aggregates.

2. **Glass:** Silica (in the form of sand) is a primary ingredient in the manufacturing of glass. It provides transparency, strength, and heat resistance to glass products such as windows, bottles, containers, and optical fibers.

Unraveling the Origins: Exploring 101 Triggers of Cancer

3. **Ceramics:** Silica is used in the production of ceramics and pottery for its ability to enhance strength, durability, and heat resistance. It's a key component in clay bodies and glazes.

4. **Paints and coatings:** Silica is used as a filler and thickening agent in paints, coatings, and sealants to improve durability, viscosity, and abrasion resistance.

5. **Cosmetics and personal care products:** Silica is commonly used in cosmetics and personal care products such as toothpaste, exfoliating scrubs, makeup foundations, and powders for its absorbent and abrasive properties.

6. **Food and beverage:** Silica is used as an anti-caking agent in powdered foods (e.g., spices, powdered drinks) to prevent clumping and improve flowability. It's also used as a filtering agent in the production of beer, wine, and edible oils.

7. **Pharmaceuticals:** Silica is used in pharmaceuticals as an excipient (inactive ingredient) in tablet formulations to improve flowability during manufacturing and to prevent caking and sticking.

8. **Electronic devices:** Silica is used in the production of silicon chips and other electronic components due to its semiconductor properties.

9. **Rubber and plastics:** Silica is added to rubber and plastic compounds to improve reinforcement, hardness, and resistance to abrasion and heat.

10. **Water filtration:** Silica-based materials are used in water filtration systems to remove impurities and improve water quality.

These are just a few examples of the many products and applications where silica is used. Its versatility and abundance make it a crucial component in various industries.

Crystalline silica particles are very small and can be inhaled deep into the lungs, where they can cause damage and inflammation over time. Prolonged or repeated exposure to respirable crystalline silica dust, especially in occupational settings where it is generated through activities like mining, quarrying, drilling, cutting, or grinding of silica-containing materials, can lead to serious health problems, including lung cancer.

The carcinogenicity of crystalline silica is primarily attributed to its ability to cause silicosis, a progressive and irreversible lung disease characterized by inflammation and scarring of lung tissue. Chronic inflammation and tissue damage increase the risk of lung cancer development. Additionally, crystalline silica particles can cause genetic mutations in lung cells, further increasing the risk of cancer.

Occupational safety organizations, such as the International Agency for Research on Cancer (IARC) and the National Institute for Occupational Safety and Health (NIOSH), have classified crystalline silica as a Group 1 carcinogen, indicating that there is sufficient evidence to support its carcinogenicity in humans. As a result, regulatory agencies have established exposure limits and guidelines to protect workers from excessive exposure to crystalline silica dust in the workplace.

Unraveling the Origins: Exploring 101 Triggers of Cancer

Trigger 49/101 – Cyclamates

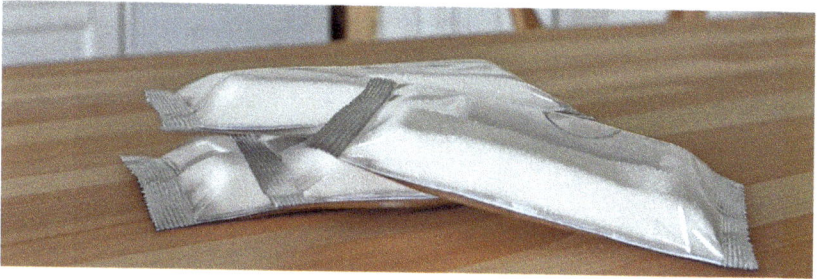

Report: IARC, Vol 22, 1980
Category: chemical
Cancer Type(s): urinary tract, bladder

Cyclamates are a type of artificial sweetener that was widely used in food and beverage products as a sugar substitute. They are derived from cyclohexylsulfamic acid and were first discovered in 1937 by Michael Sveda, a chemist working at the University of Illinois.

Cyclamates are highly sweet, often described as being around 30 to 50 times sweeter than sucrose (table sugar), making them an attractive option for reducing calorie intake in foods and beverages intended for people with diabetes or those seeking to control their sugar consumption. They were commonly used in various products such as soft drinks, tabletop sweeteners, desserts, and other low-calorie or sugar-free items.

However, concerns about the safety of cyclamates emerged in the late 1960s and early 1970s. Studies conducted on laboratory animals suggested a potential link between cyclamate consumption and bladder cancer. As a result, cyclamates were banned in several countries, including the United States, Canada, and the European Union.

While cyclamates remain legal and in use in some countries, their popularity has declined significantly in favor of other artificial sweeteners like aspartame, sucralose, and stevia, which have not raised the same level of safety concerns. Despite the ban in some regions, cyclamates continue to be a topic of scientific research and debate regarding their safety and potential health effects.

Cyclamates were once widely used as artificial sweeteners in various food and beverage products, particularly those marketed as low-calorie or sugar-free alternatives. Some common products that may have contained cyclamates in the past include:

1. **Soft drinks:** Diet or sugar-free soft drinks, including colas, fruit-flavored sodas, and other carbonated beverages, often used cyclamates as a sweetening agent to reduce calorie content.

2. **Tabletop sweeteners:** Cyclamate-based sweeteners were commonly used in packets or tablets as a sugar substitute for coffee, tea, and other beverages, as well as for sprinkling on cereals or fruits.

3. **Desserts and confectionery:** Sugar-free desserts, such as puddings, gelatin desserts, and ice cream, may have been sweetened with cyclamates. Additionally, some sugar-free candies and chewing gums may have contained cyclamates.

4. **Preserves and condiments:** Certain jams, jellies, syrups, and sauces may have used cyclamates to provide sweetness without added sugars.

5. **Baked goods:** Some low-calorie or sugar-free baked goods, including cakes, cookies, and pastries, may have been sweetened with cyclamates.

Unraveling the Origins: Exploring 101 Triggers of Cancer

However, it's important to note that the use of cyclamates has been banned or heavily restricted in many countries due to safety concerns, particularly regarding potential carcinogenicity. As a result, their use in food and beverage products has declined significantly over the years.

Here are some key reasons why cyclamates were considered carcinogenic:

1. **Metabolism in the body:** When consumed, cyclamate is metabolized in the body into cyclohexylamine, which has been implicated in bladder cancer development in animal studies. Cyclohexylamine can react with nitrites in the body to form N-nitrosocyclohexylamine, a compound that is known to be carcinogenic.

2. **Bladder toxicity:** Studies showed that high doses of cyclamates led to bladder stones and hyperplasia (abnormal cell growth) in the bladders of rats, which are considered precursors to cancer. The formation of bladder stones may have contributed to chronic irritation and inflammation, increasing the risk of cancer development.

3. **Genotoxicity:** Cyclamate and its metabolites have been found to exhibit genotoxic effects, meaning they can damage DNA and potentially lead to mutations that contribute to cancer development.

Due to these concerns, regulatory agencies in many countries, including the United States, Canada, and the European Union, decided to ban or severely restrict the use of cyclamates as a food additive. However, it's important to note that the carcinogenicity of cyclamates remains a topic of scientific debate, and some countries still permit their use in specific products under certain conditions.

Trigger 50/101 – Diethylstilbestrol

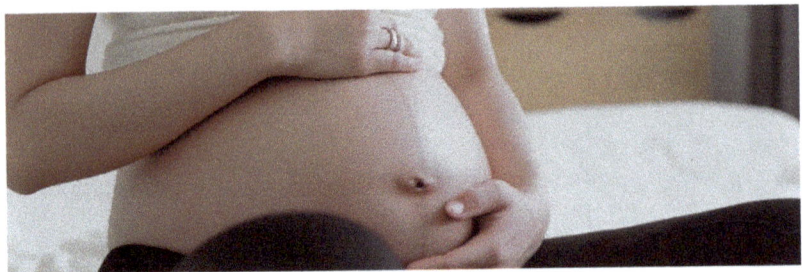

Report: 1st Report on Carcinogens
Category: chemical
Cancer Type(s): mammary, cervix, testicular

Diethylstilbestrol (DES) is a synthetic estrogen that was first synthesized in 1938. It was prescribed to pregnant women between the late 1930s and early 1970s to prevent miscarriages, premature labor, and other pregnancy complications. DES was also sometimes given to livestock to promote growth.

However, in the early 1970s, DES was discovered to be associated with a range of serious health issues in both the women who took it during pregnancy and their offspring. These health effects included an increased risk of reproductive tract abnormalities, infertility, and a rare form of vaginal cancer (clear cell adenocarcinoma) in daughters exposed to DES in utero. Sons of women who took DES during pregnancy may also have an increased risk of certain health problems, such as genital abnormalities and testicular cancer.

As a result of these findings, the use of DES during pregnancy was discontinued in many countries, and regulatory agencies issued warnings against its use. However, the long-term health effects of DES exposure continue to be studied, as individuals who were exposed in utero may experience health issues later in life.

Unraveling the Origins: Exploring 101 Triggers of Cancer

Despite its risks, DES has also been used in some medical treatments, such as hormone therapy for certain types of cancer, though its use in these contexts has become increasingly rare due to safety concerns and the availability of alternative treatments.

Diethylstilbestrol (DES) was used in the past as a growth promoter in livestock, including cattle, to increase weight gain and improve feed efficiency. However, due to concerns about its carcinogenicity and other health risks, its use has been banned in many countries for several decades.

In the United States, the Food and Drug Administration (FDA) banned DES for use in cattle feed in 1979. Similarly, the use of DES in livestock has been prohibited in the European Union and many other countries.

Diethylstilbestrol (DES) is classified as a carcinogen because of its ability to disrupt normal hormonal function in the body, particularly its estrogenic effects. DES is a synthetic estrogen, and exposure to high levels of estrogenic compounds has been linked to an increased risk of certain cancers.

The carcinogenicity of DES primarily stems from its ability to act as an endocrine disruptor, mimicking the effects of natural estrogen hormones in the body. This can lead to various cellular changes and disruptions in hormonal balance, which may promote the development of cancerous cells.

Furthermore, while less studied, there is also some evidence suggesting that sons of women who took DES during pregnancy may have an increased risk of testicular cancer and other health issues related to reproductive tract abnormalities.

Trigger 51/101 – Dimethylcarbamoyl Chloride

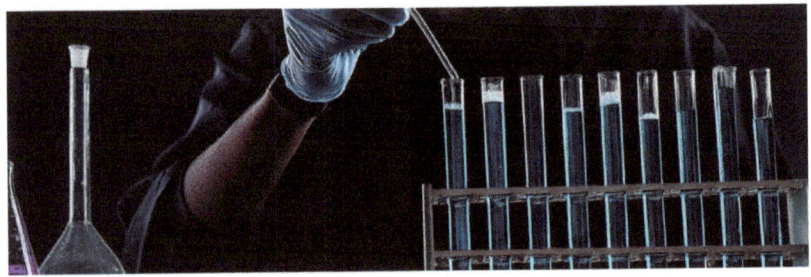

Report: 2nd Report on Carcinogens
Category: chemical
Cancer Type(s): skin, nasal

Dimethylcarbamoyl chloride (DMCC) is primarily used as a reagent(compound added to a system to cause a chemical reaction) in organic synthesis, particularly in the pharmaceutical and agrochemical industries. It is a versatile compound that serves as a key building block in the production of various pharmaceuticals, pesticides, and other specialty chemicals. One of the most common applications of dimethylcarbamoyl chloride is in the synthesis of carbamates, which are important intermediates in the production of insecticides, herbicides, and fungicides. It is also used in the preparation of pharmaceuticals, such as certain antibiotics and antihistamines.

Due to its reactive nature and potential hazards, dimethylcarbamoyl chloride should be handled with care by trained professionals in a controlled laboratory environment, using appropriate safety precautions and protective equipment.

DMCC is an alkylating agent, meaning it can add alkyl groups to DNA. This can result in DNA damage, including mutations that can disrupt normal cellular processes and lead to uncontrolled cell growth (cancer). DMCC can form adducts with DNA. DNA adducts are segments of DNA bound to a cancer-causing chemical. If these

Unraveling the Origins: Exploring 101 Triggers of Cancer

adducts are not repaired, they can result in permanent mutations during DNA replication. Studies have shown that exposure to DMCC leads to cancer in laboratory animals. These studies provide a strong basis for its classification as a carcinogen.

Some specific products and compounds that may involve the use of DMCC in their synthesis include:

1. Acetazolamide (used to treat glaucoma, epilepsy, and altitude sickness)
2. Carbachol (used to treat glaucoma and to induce miosis during ophthalmic surgery)
3. Atenolol (used to treat high blood pressure and angina)
4. Diphenhydramine (an antihistamine used to relieve symptoms of allergy, hay fever, and the common cold)
5. Aldicarb (a carbamate insecticide used to control nematodes, mites, and insects)
6. Carbaryl (a carbamate insecticide and molluscicide used to control pests in agriculture and forestry)

These examples illustrate the diverse range of products and compounds that may involve the use of DMCC as an intermediate in their synthesis. However, it's important to note that DMCC is primarily used in industrial settings and laboratory environments rather than being directly incorporated into consumer products.

Trigger 52/101 – 1,2-Dimethylhydrazine

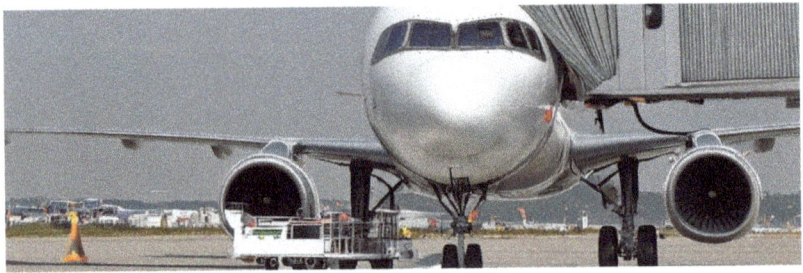

Report: 4th Report on Carcinogens
Category: chemical
Cancer Type(s): kidney, lungs, liver

1,2-Dimethylhydrazine is used primarily as a component of jet and rocket fuels, and as a plant growth control agent, In laboratory research, 1,2-dimethylhydrazine (DMH) may be used as a chemical reagent or precursor in various experiments or investigations. While its use is relatively limited due to its toxic and hazardous nature, there are some specific areas of research where DMH or its derivatives may find application:

1. **Chemical synthesis:** DMH can be used in organic synthesis as a building block or starting material for the preparation of various organic compounds. It can undergo reactions with other chemicals to introduce functional groups or modify chemical structures, allowing researchers to explore new compounds or study specific chemical reactions.

2. **Cancer research:** Despite its carcinogenic properties, DMH is sometimes used in laboratory studies involving animal models of cancer. Researchers may administer DMH to laboratory animals to induce colon or other types of cancer for studying disease mechanisms, treatment strategies, or the effects of potential anticancer agents.

3. **Toxicology studies:** DMH may be used in toxicology research to investigate its acute or chronic effects on biological systems. Researchers may expose cells, tissues, or organisms to DMH to study its toxicity mechanisms, determine safe exposure limits, or evaluate potential antidotes or treatments for DMH poisoning.

4. **Environmental research:** DMH and its derivatives may be studied in environmental research to assess their presence, fate, and potential impact in the environment. Researchers may investigate DMH contamination in soil, water, or air, as well as its interactions with living organisms and ecosystems.

It's important to note that the use of DMH in laboratory research requires careful handling and appropriate safety precautions due to its toxic and hazardous properties. Researchers working with DMH should adhere to established safety guidelines and protocols to minimize exposure risks and ensure the safety of laboratory personnel and the surrounding environment.
Specific laboratory studies involving 1,2-dimethylhydrazine (DMH) or its derivatives may include:

1. **Colon cancer induction studies:** DMH is commonly used in laboratory research to induce colon cancer in animal models, particularly rodents. Researchers administer DMH to experimental animals to study the development, progression, and treatment of colon cancer. These studies may involve investigating the molecular mechanisms of carcinogenesis, evaluating potential preventive or therapeutic interventions, and assessing the efficacy of anticancer drugs.

2. **Toxicity testing:** DMH is used in toxicology studies to assess its acute and chronic toxicity in various biological systems. Researchers may expose cells, tissues, or organisms to different concentrations of DMH to determine its effects on

cell viability, organ function, and overall health. These studies help to establish safe exposure limits, identify potential health hazards, and develop strategies for mitigating DMH toxicity.

3. **Mechanistic studies:** Researchers may use DMH in mechanistic studies to investigate the underlying mechanisms of its carcinogenicity and toxic effects. This may involve exploring the biochemical, molecular, and cellular pathways involved in DMH-induced carcinogenesis, genotoxicity, and oxidative stress. Understanding these mechanisms is essential for developing targeted interventions and preventive measures.

4. **Pharmacokinetic studies:** Pharmacokinetic studies involve investigating the absorption, distribution, metabolism, and excretion of DMH in living organisms. Researchers may administer DMH to experimental animals and analyze blood, tissue, or urine samples to determine its pharmacokinetic properties and biodistribution. These studies provide valuable insights into DMH metabolism and toxicity mechanisms.

5. **Environmental fate and transport studies:** In environmental research, DMH may be used in laboratory studies to investigate its fate, transport, and degradation in different environmental compartments. Researchers may simulate environmental conditions and assess the persistence, transformation, and bioaccumulation of DMH in soil, water, sediments, and biota. These studies help to assess environmental risks and develop strategies for environmental remediation.

Overall, laboratory studies involving DMH play a critical role in advancing our understanding of its carcinogenicity, toxicity, and environmental impact, as well as informing regulatory decisions and public health policies related to its use and exposure.

Unraveling the Origins: Exploring 101 Triggers of Cancer

Trigger 53/101 – Dimethylvinyl Chloride

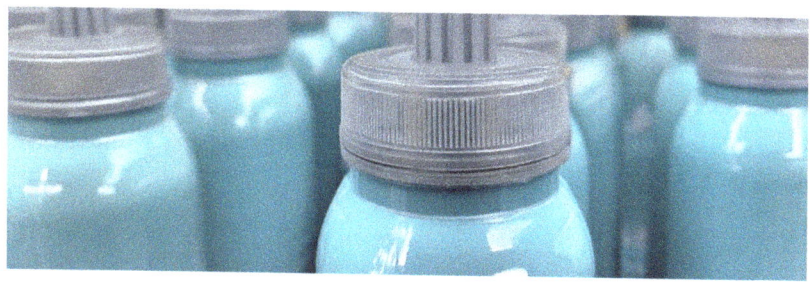

Report: 6th Report on Carcinogens
Category: chemical
Cancer Type(s): forestomach, nasal, oral-cavity, papilloma

Dimethylvinyl chloride is primarily used as a chemical intermediate in organic synthesis. It can undergo various chemical reactions to produce other compounds or polymers with specific properties.

Some specific functional materials that may incorporate DMVC-derived polymers or copolymers include:

1. **Coatings:** DMVC-derived polymers or copolymers may be used in the formulation of coatings for applications such as paints, varnishes, and protective coatings. These coatings may offer properties such as adhesion, durability, chemical resistance, and weatherability.

2. **Adhesives:** DMVC-based polymers or copolymers can be used in the formulation of adhesives and sealants for bonding various substrates in construction, automotive, packaging, and other industries. These adhesives may provide properties such as high strength, flexibility, and heat resistance.

3. **Membranes:** DMVC-derived polymers or copolymers may be used in the fabrication of membranes for separation processes, such as reverse osmosis, ultrafiltration, and gas separation. These membranes may exhibit properties such as high permeability, selectivity, and chemical resistance.

4. **Packaging materials:** DMVC-based polymers or copolymers may be used in the production of packaging materials such as films, sheets, and containers. These materials may offer properties such as barrier properties, transparency, flexibility, and heat sealability.

5. **Textiles:** DMVC-derived polymers or copolymers may be incorporated into textiles and fibers to impart specific properties such as flame retardancy, water repellency, and antistatic properties.

6. **Electronic materials:** DMVC-based polymers or copolymers may find applications in electronic materials such as printed circuit boards, encapsulants, and conductive coatings. These materials may offer properties such as electrical insulation, thermal conductivity, and flame retardancy.

7. **Biomedical materials:** DMVC-derived polymers or copolymers may be used in biomedical applications such as drug delivery systems, tissue engineering scaffolds, and medical implants. These materials may exhibit properties such as biocompatibility, biodegradability, and controlled release of drugs or bioactive molecules.

8. **Orthopedic implants:** Polymers derived from DMVC may be used in orthopedic implants such as joint prostheses (e.g., hip or knee implants), bone plates, screws, and spinal implants. These implants may be made from polymer materials with

properties such as biocompatibility, mechanical strength, and wear resistance.

9. **Dental implants:** Dental implants are used to replace missing teeth and provide support for dental prostheses such as crowns, bridges, and dentures. Polymer materials derived from DMVC may be used in dental implant components such as abutments, healing caps, and implant coatings to enhance biocompatibility and tissue integration.

10. **Cardiovascular implants:** Polymer coatings derived from DMVC may be applied to cardiovascular implants such as stents, vascular grafts, and heart valves to improve biocompatibility, reduce thrombogenicity, and prevent restenosis or thrombosis.

11. **Soft tissue implants:** Polymers derived from DMVC may be used in soft tissue implants such as breast implants, facial implants, and tissue fillers. These implants may be made from biocompatible polymer materials that mimic the properties of natural tissues and provide aesthetic or reconstructive benefits.

12. **Neurological implants:** Polymer materials derived from DMVC may be used in neurological implants such as electrodes, neural probes, and deep brain stimulation devices. These implants may be coated with biocompatible polymer materials to improve tissue compatibility and reduce inflammatory responses.

It's important to note that the selection of materials for medical implants is subject to rigorous testing and regulatory approval to ensure safety, efficacy, and biocompatibility. The specific choice of polymer materials, including those derived from DMVC, depends on factors such as the intended application, implant design, mechanical requirements, and biocompatibility considerations.

Trigger 54/101 – N,N-Dimethyl-p-toluidine

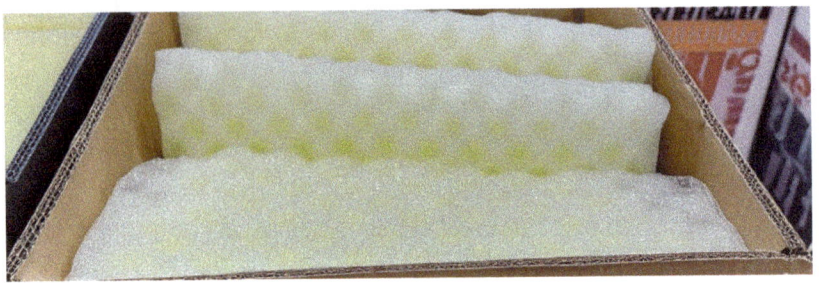

Report: NTP Technical Report CAS No. 99-997-8
Category: chemical
Cancer Type(s): nose, thyroid, stomach

N,N-Dimethyl-p-toluidine also known as DMT or DMP-T, is commonly used as a catalyst or curing agent in various industrial applications, particularly in the production of polyurethane foams, coatings, adhesives, and resins. It serves as a promoter in the polymerization or cross-linking reactions of certain polymers, helping to accelerate the curing process and improve the mechanical properties of the final products.

In addition to its use in industrial applications, N,N-Dimethyl-p-toluidine may also find use in laboratory research, particularly in organic synthesis or as a reagent in chemical reactions.

However, it's important to note that N,N-Dimethyl-p-toluidine is considered hazardous, and exposure to it should be minimized. It can be harmful if inhaled, absorbed through the skin, or ingested, and prolonged or repeated exposure may cause adverse health effects. Therefore, appropriate safety precautions, such as proper ventilation and personal protective equipment, should be followed when handling this compound.

Some specific products in which DMT may be used include:

1. **Polyurethane foams:** DMT is commonly used as a curing agent or catalyst in the production of polyurethane foams, which are widely used in applications such as insulation, cushioning, and packaging. It helps to initiate and accelerate the polymerization reaction between polyols and isocyanates, leading to the formation of the foam structure.

2. **Coatings and paints:** DMT may be used as a curing agent or promoter in the formulation of coatings and paints for applications such as automotive finishes, industrial coatings, and architectural paints. It helps to cross-link the polymer chains, improve the adhesion and durability of the coatings, and enhance their resistance to chemicals, weathering, and abrasion.

3. **Adhesives and sealants:** DMT can serve as a curing agent or promoter in the production of adhesives and sealants used in construction, automotive, aerospace, and other industries. It helps to initiate the polymerization or cross-linking reactions, leading to the formation of strong and durable bonds between substrates.

4. **Resins and composites:** DMT may be used as a curing agent or catalyst in the production of resins and composites, such as epoxy resins, polyester resins, and acrylic resins. It helps to promote the curing or cross-linking of the resin matrix, improving the mechanical properties, heat resistance, and chemical resistance of the final products.

5. **Polymer additives:** DMT-derived compounds may be used as additives in polymer formulations to modify the processing or performance properties of the polymers. For example, they may act as chain extenders, cross-linking agents, or reactive diluents to tailor the viscosity, rheology, or cure kinetics of the polymers.

Overall, DMT and its derivatives play a crucial role in the formulation and production of a wide range of industrial products, contributing to their performance, durability, and versatility in various applications.

N,N-Dimethyl-p-toluidine (DMT) is classified as a potential carcinogen due to its association with cancer in laboratory animals and its potential to cause adverse health effects in humans. Several factors contribute to its carcinogenicity:

Overall, the carcinogenicity of DMT is supported by evidence from experimental studies in animals, mechanistic studies elucidating its genotoxic and tumorigenic effects, and epidemiological observations of increased cancer risk associated with exposure to aromatic amines. As a result, DMT is classified as a potential human carcinogen by regulatory agencies such as the International Agency for Research on Cancer (IARC).

Unraveling the Origins: Exploring 101 Triggers of Cancer

Trigger 55/101 – 1,4-Dioxane

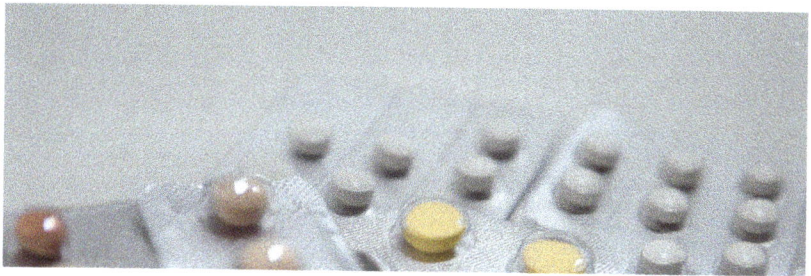

Report: 2nd Report on Carcinogens
Category: chemical
Cancer Type(s): livery, nasal, mammary, kidney

1,4-Dioxane, often referred to simply as dioxane, is a heterocyclic organic compound primarily used as a solvent in various industrial and laboratory applications, including:

1. **Chemical synthesis:** Dioxane is commonly used as a solvent in organic synthesis reactions to dissolve and facilitate the reaction of various organic compounds. It is particularly useful in reactions that involve polar and nonpolar compounds or in reactions that require elevated temperatures.

2. **Extraction:** Dioxane is used as a solvent for the extraction of natural products, such as plant extracts or essential oils, in industries such as pharmaceuticals, cosmetics, and flavors and fragrances.

3. **Polymer processing:** Dioxane is used as a solvent in the processing of certain polymers, resins, and plastics, particularly in the production of cellulose acetate, cellulose ethers, and polyurethanes.

4. **Cleaning and degreasing:** Dioxane is used as a solvent in cleaning and degreasing applications, such as in the cleaning of metal parts or electronic components, due to its ability to dissolve a wide range of organic compounds.

5. **Laboratory research:** Dioxane is used as a solvent in laboratory research for various applications, including chromatography, spectroscopy, and synthesis of organic compounds. It is particularly valued for its ability to dissolve both polar and nonpolar compounds.

6. **Cosmetics and personal care products:** Dioxane may be used as a solvent or as an ingredient in cosmetics and personal care products, such as lotions, creams, shampoos, and soaps. It can function as a solvent for fragrances, dyes, or other active ingredients.

While dioxane has many industrial applications, it is also considered a contaminant of concern due to its potential health and environmental risks. It is classified as a probable human carcinogen by the International Agency for Research on Cancer (IARC) based on animal studies showing carcinogenic effects. Therefore, efforts are made to minimize exposure to dioxane and to control its release into the environment.

It's important to note that while 1,4-dioxane may be used in the production of these products, it is typically removed or present only in trace amounts in the final consumer products due to regulatory requirements and quality control measures aimed at minimizing its presence. Nonetheless, exposure to 1,4-dioxane can occur through inhalation, skin contact, or ingestion, particularly in occupational settings or with prolonged use of certain products, which has raised concerns about its potential health risks.

1,4-Dioxane is not typically used as an active ingredient in medications. Instead, it may be used as a solvent or as part of the manufacturing process for certain pharmaceuticals. Its use in pharmaceuticals is primarily as a solvent in the synthesis or formulation of medications rather than as a direct component of the final product.

Some medications that may involve the use of 1,4-dioxane in their production process include:

1. **Tablets and capsules:** 1,4-Dioxane may be used as a solvent in the synthesis of active pharmaceutical ingredients (APIs) or in the formulation of tablets, capsules, or other solid dosage forms. It helps dissolve and process the various components of the medication to create a uniform and stable product.

2. **Liquid formulations:** In liquid medications such as solutions, suspensions, or syrups, 1,4-dioxane may be used as a solvent to dissolve the active ingredients or other components of the formulation. It aids in the solubilization and dispersion of the ingredients to ensure proper dosing and administration.

3. **Topical preparations:** Some topical medications, such as creams, lotions, or ointments, may contain 1,4-dioxane as a solvent or as part of the formulation. It helps dissolve the active ingredients and other components of the preparation to create a consistent and effective product for application to the skin.

It's important to note that while 1,4-dioxane may be used in the production process of certain medications, regulatory agencies typically require manufacturers to ensure that residual levels of 1,4-dioxane in the final pharmaceutical products are within acceptable limits. This is done to minimize potential exposure and ensure the safety of the medications for consumers. Therefore, the presence of 1,4-dioxane in pharmaceutical products, if present at all, is usually at very low concentrations and is tightly regulated.

Trigger 56/101 – Epichlorohydrin

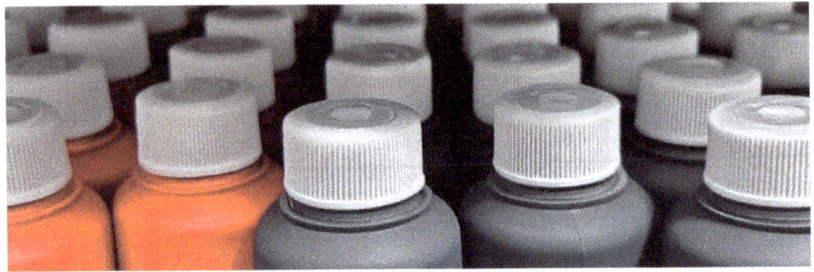

Report: 4th Report on Carcinogens
Category: chemical
Cancer Type(s): stomach, nasal cavity

Epichlorohydrin is primarily used in the production of epoxy resins, which are versatile polymers widely used in various applications such as adhesives, coatings, composites, and electronics.

Some key properties and uses of epichlorohydrin include:

1. **Epoxy resin production:** The most significant use of epichlorohydrin is as a precursor in the synthesis of epoxy resins. These resins have excellent adhesive properties, chemical resistance, and mechanical strength, making them valuable in a wide range of industrial and consumer applications.

2. **Other chemical synthesis:** Epichlorohydrin is also used as an intermediate in the production of various chemicals, including glycerol, plastics, pharmaceuticals, and water treatment chemicals. It can undergo reactions such as hydrolysis, chlorination, and oxidation to yield different compounds with diverse applications.

3. **Solvent:** In addition to its role as a precursor in chemical synthesis, epichlorohydrin can also function as a solvent for various organic compounds. It is soluble in common organic solvents and is used in certain industrial processes and formulations where its solvent properties are beneficial.

4. **Water treatment:** Epichlorohydrin is sometimes used in water treatment applications as a biocide or disinfectant to control microbial growth and pathogens in water systems. However, its use in this capacity is limited due to its toxicity and environmental concerns.

5. **Coatings:** Epoxy coatings are used to protect and enhance the appearance of surfaces in consumer products and structures. They are applied to floors, countertops, tabletops, and other surfaces to provide a durable, seamless finish that is resistant to abrasion, chemicals, and stains. Epoxy coatings are popular in home renovation projects and commercial settings.

6. **Electronics:** Epoxy resins are used in the manufacturing of electronic components and devices, including printed circuit boards (PCBs), semiconductors, and encapsulation materials for electronic assemblies. They provide insulation, protection, and mechanical support for sensitive electronic components, helping to ensure reliability and longevity.

Overall, while epichlorohydrin itself is not directly used in consumer products, the epoxy resins derived from it have numerous consumer applications in adhesives, coatings, sealants, composite materials, and electronics, among others. These consumer products benefit from the unique properties of epoxy resins, including their strength, durability, and versatility. Epichlorohydrin is classified as a potential carcinogen based on studies that have shown an increased risk of cancer associated with exposure to this chemical. Several factors contribute to its classification as a carcinogen:

Trigger 57/101 – Erionite

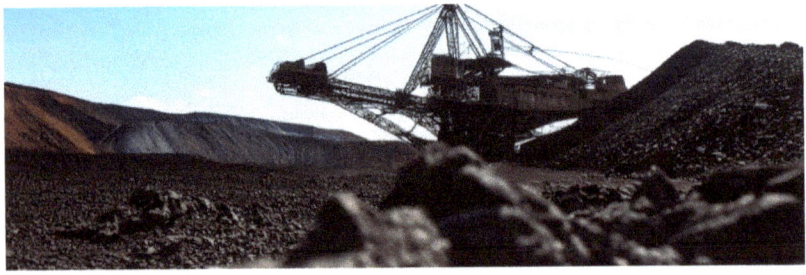

Report: 7th Report on Carcinogens
Category: chemical
Cancer Type(s): mesothelioma, lung

Erionite is a naturally occurring mineral, is known for its fibrous or needle-like crystal morphology and its high surface area, which make it useful in various industrial applications. Erionite is found in volcanic rocks and sedimentary deposits that have undergone alteration by hydrothermal fluids. It is most commonly associated with volcanic tuffs, basalts, and sedimentary rocks rich in zeolitic minerals.

Due to its high surface area and cation exchange capacity, erionite has potential applications in industries such as water purification,

Unraveling the Origins: Exploring 101 Triggers of Cancer

gas adsorption, catalysis, and ion exchange. Zeolites, including erionite, have been studied as additives in concrete and construction materials to improve properties such as strength, durability, and moisture resistance. Erionite's pozzolanic properties may contribute to the enhancement of concrete performance, although its use in construction materials is limited due to concerns about potential health risks associated with exposure to respirable fibers.

Like other fibrous minerals, erionite poses potential health risks if inhaled as respirable fibers. Chronic exposure to airborne erionite fibers has been associated with the development of respiratory diseases, including mesothelioma, lung cancer, and other lung disorders. Erionite exposure is of particular concern in areas where natural deposits are present and may become airborne through mining, construction, or other human activities.

Erionite health hazards, particularly its association with respiratory diseases, underscore the importance of understanding and mitigating exposure risks in occupational and environmental settings.

Trigger 58/101 – Ethylbenzene

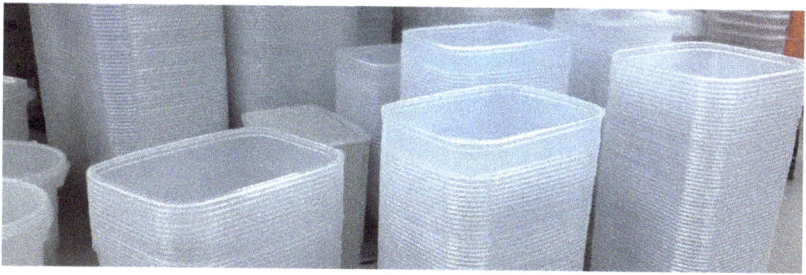

Report: NIH Publication No. 99-3956
Category: chemical
Cancer Type(s): kidneys, testes, head

Ethylbenzene is one of the largest volume chemicals produced globally and is commonly used as a precursor in the production of styrene, which is used to make polystyrene plastics and synthetic rubber. Ethylbenzene is also used as a solvent in the manufacturing of coatings, paints, varnishes, and adhesives. Additionally, it is used as an intermediate in the synthesis of other chemicals, including phenylethanol, diethylbenzene, and acetophenone.

Ethylbenzene can pose health risks if inhaled or ingested in large quantities. Acute exposure to ethylbenzene vapor can cause irritation of the respiratory tract, eyes, and skin. Prolonged or repeated exposure may lead to central nervous system effects, such as headache, dizziness, nausea, and in severe cases, unconsciousness or death. Chronic exposure to ethylbenzene has been associated with potential adverse effects on the liver, kidneys, and blood-forming tissues.

Ethylbenzene is released into the environment during its production, use, and disposal. It can contaminate soil, water, and air through industrial emissions, spills, and improper disposal practices. Ethylbenzene is persistent in the environment and may undergo biodegradation over time. However, it can accumulate in aquatic organisms and may pose risks to ecosystems and human health through the food chain.

Overall, ethylbenzene is an industrial chemical with widespread use as a precursor in the production of styrene and as a solvent in various applications. However, it is essential to handle ethylbenzene with care and implement appropriate safety measures to minimize health and environmental risks associated with its use.

Ethylbenzene has been shown to exhibit genotoxic effects in laboratory studies, meaning it can damage DNA and potentially lead to mutations and chromosomal abnormalities that contribute to cancer development.

Trigger 59/101 – Ethylene Oxide (EO)

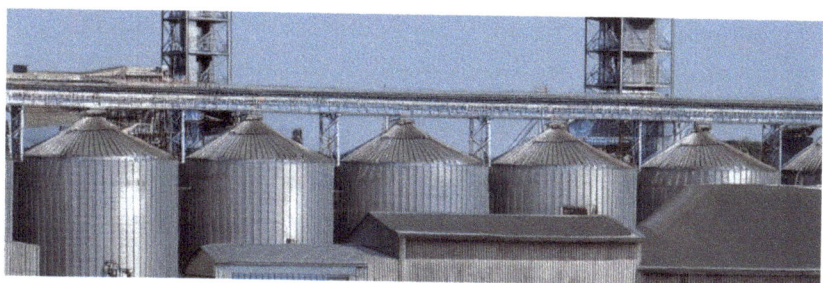

Report: 4th Report on Carcinogens
Category: chemical
Cancer Type(s): lymphoma and leukemia

Ethylene oxide is used in a wide range of industrial and commercial applications due to its versatile properties.

Some common uses of ethylene oxide include:

1. Sterilization: Ethylene oxide is widely used as a sterilizing agent for medical devices, pharmaceuticals, and other heat-sensitive materials. It penetrates packaging materials and kills microorganisms, including bacteria, viruses, and spores, making it suitable for sterilizing a wide range of medical and healthcare products.

2. Chemical synthesis: Ethylene oxide is used as a raw material or intermediate in the production of various chemicals, including ethylene glycol (used in antifreeze and polyester resins), surfactants, glycol ethers, ethanolamines, and polyethylene

glycols (PEGs). It serves as a building block for synthesizing complex organic compounds in the chemical industry.

3. Fumigation: Ethylene oxide is sometimes used as a fumigant for disinfecting and pest control in agricultural and food processing facilities. It can penetrate porous materials and kill insects, fungi, and other pests without leaving residues, making it suitable for treating stored grains, spices, and other commodities.

Ethylene oxide is classified as a carcinogen by several regulatory agencies, including the International Agency for Research on Cancer (IARC) and the U.S. Environmental Protection Agency (EPA). Prolonged or repeated exposure to ethylene oxide vapor has been associated with an increased risk of cancer, particularly leukemia, lymphoma, and breast cancer. Ethylene oxide is also a potent irritant to the respiratory tract and skin and can cause adverse health effects, including nausea, headache, dizziness, and respiratory symptoms, at high concentrations.

Overall, while ethylene oxide is a valuable chemical with numerous industrial applications, its potential health hazards underscore the importance of handling and using it with care and implementing appropriate safety measures to protect human health and the environment.

Unraveling the Origins: Exploring 101 Triggers of Cancer

Trigger 60/101 – Etoposide

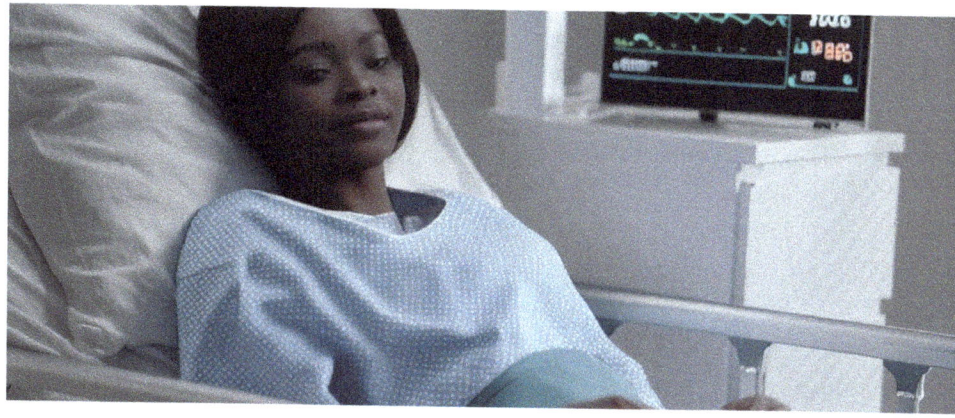

Report: NTP. Etoposide (33419-42-0)
Category: chemical
Cancer Type(s): acute myeloid leukemia, non-hodgkin lymphoma

Etoposide is a chemotherapy medication used primarily in the treatment of various types of cancer. It belongs to a class of drugs known as topoisomerase inhibitors, which interfere with the action of enzymes called topoisomerases. These enzymes are involved in the unwinding and rewinding of DNA during cell division, making them essential for DNA replication and repair.

Here are some of the cancer treatments it's used for:

1. Small cell lung cancer: Etoposide is often used in combination with other chemotherapy drugs, such as cisplatin or carboplatin, as a first-line treatment for small cell lung cancer.

2. Testicular cancer: Etoposide is part of the standard chemotherapy regimen for treating testicular cancer, usually in combination with other drugs like cisplatin and bleomycin.

3. Lymphomas: Etoposide may be used in the treatment of certain types of lymphomas, such as Hodgkin lymphoma and non-Hodgkin lymphoma, either as part of a combination chemotherapy regimen or as a single agent.

4. Leukemias: Etoposide is sometimes used in the treatment of acute myeloid leukemia (AML) and acute lymphoblastic leukemia (ALL), particularly in combination with other chemotherapy drugs.

Certain chemotherapy drugs, including etoposide, can increase the risk of developing secondary cancers as a potential long-term side effect of treatment. This increased risk is primarily due to the DNA-damaging effects of chemotherapy on healthy cells, which can sometimes lead to mutations that contribute to the development of new cancers.

Chemotherapy drugs like etoposide work by targeting rapidly dividing cells, including cancer cells, but they can also affect normal cells in the body. While the primary goal of chemotherapy is to kill cancer cells, some healthy cells, particularly those with high rates of proliferation, may also be damaged in the process. Over time, this damage can potentially increase the risk of genetic mutations and the development of secondary cancers, although the overall benefits of chemotherapy in treating the primary cancer generally outweigh this risk.

The specific risk of developing secondary cancers as a result of chemotherapy treatment varies depending on factors such as the type of cancer being treated, the specific chemotherapy drugs used, the dose and duration of treatment, and individual patient factors. Some types of secondary cancers associated with chemotherapy treatment include leukemia, myelodysplastic syndrome (MDS), and certain solid tumors.

Unraveling the Origins: Exploring 101 Triggers of Cancer

Trigger 61/101 – Hexachloro-1,3-butadiene

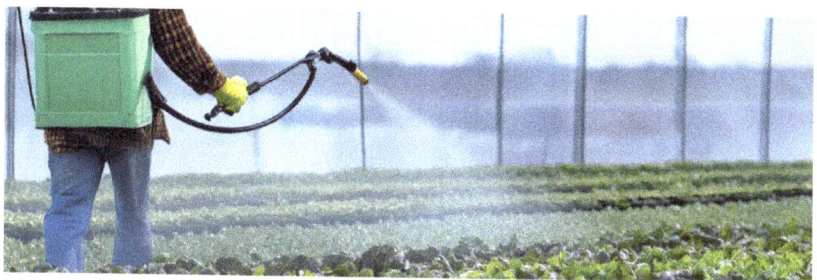

Report: NIH Publication No. 991-3120
Category: chemical
Cancer Type(s): kidney

Hexachloro-1,3-butadiene, also known as HCBD, is a synthetic chemical compound belonging to the class of chlorinated hydrocarbons. It is derived from butadiene, a colorless gas commonly used in the production of synthetic rubber and plastics.

Here are some key points about hexachloro-1,3-butadiene:

1. HCBD was historically used as an intermediate chemical in the production of various products, including pesticides, herbicides, and flame retardants. It was also used as a solvent in chemical synthesis and as a component in hydraulic fluids and lubricants. However, many uses of HCBD have been phased out or restricted due to environmental and health concerns.

2. **Health and environmental effects:** HCBD is classified as a probable human carcinogen by the International Agency for Research on Cancer (IARC) based on limited evidence from animal studies. Chronic exposure to HCBD has been associated

with adverse effects on the liver, kidneys, and central nervous system in animals. HCBD is also persistent in the environment and can bioaccumulate in aquatic organisms, posing risks to ecosystems.

3. **Regulatory status:** HCBD is regulated by various environmental and health agencies due to its potential hazards. It is listed as a hazardous air pollutant under the U.S. Clean Air Act and is subject to regulation under other environmental laws and regulations in many countries. Efforts to reduce emissions and minimize exposure to HCBD are ongoing to protect human health and the environment.

Trigger 62/101 – Indium Phosphide

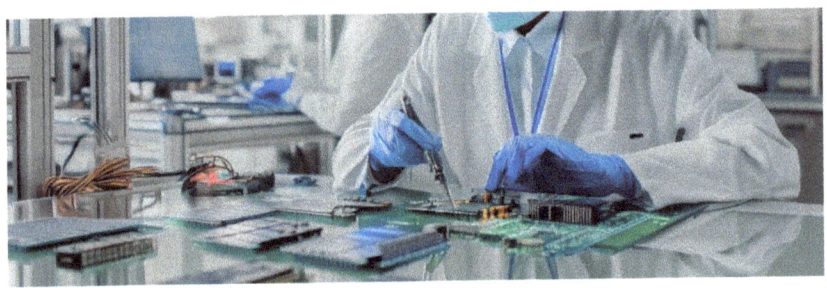

Report: NTP CAS NO. 22398-80-7
Category: chemical
Cancer Type(s): lung, colon

Indium phosphide (InP) is a semiconductor compound. Indium phosphide exhibits several favorable properties for semiconductor applications, including a direct bandgap energy of approximately 1.35 electron volts (eV) at room temperature, high electron mobility, and high thermal conductivity. These properties make it suitable for use in optoelectronic and electronic devices operating in the infrared region of the electromagnetic spectrum.

1. **Optoelectronic applications:** Indium phosphide is widely used in the fabrication of optoelectronic devices, such as light-emitting diodes (LEDs), laser diodes, photodetectors, and optical modulators. InP-based devices are commonly employed in telecommunications, fiber-optic communications, optical sensing, and high-speed data transmission applications due to their efficient light emission and detection properties.

2. **Electronic applications:** Indium phosphide is used in the manufacture of high-frequency electronic devices, such as heterojunction bipolar transistors (HBTs) and high-electron-mobility transistors (HEMTs). These devices leverage the high electron mobility of indium phosphide to achieve high-speed performance and low noise operation, making them suitable for applications in microwave and millimeter-wave communication systems, radar systems, and wireless networks.

3. **Research and development:** Indium phosphide continues to be the subject of research and development efforts aimed at improving device performance, reducing production costs, and expanding its range of applications. Researchers are exploring novel device structures, materials integration techniques, and growth methods to enhance the efficiency, reliability, and scalability of indium phosphide-based devices.

4. **Industry and commercialization:** Indium phosphide is produced and supplied by semiconductor manufacturers and materials suppliers worldwide. It is a critical material in the semiconductor industry and plays a key role in the development of advanced optoelectronic and electronic

technologies. InP-based devices are commercially available from various vendors and are used in a wide range of applications across telecommunications, data communications, aerospace, defense, and healthcare sectors.

Indium compounds, particularly certain soluble forms such as indium tin oxide (ITO) used in the electronics industry, have raised health concerns due to their potential to cause lung damage and, in some cases, lung cancer. These concerns primarily arise from occupational exposures in industries where indium compounds are used or processed, such as semiconductor manufacturing, indium plating, and indium reclaiming.

Exposure to indium compounds, particularly through inhalation of indium-containing dust or fumes, can lead to the development of pulmonary diseases such as indium lung disease and interstitial lung fibrosis. These conditions are characterized by inflammation and scarring of lung tissue, which can impair lung function and increase the risk of respiratory complications, including lung cancer.

Trigger 63/101 – Isoprene

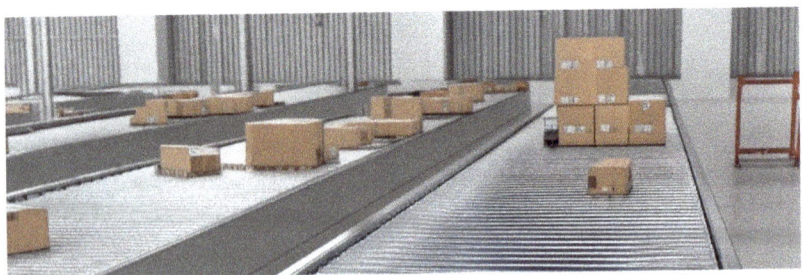

Report: 15th Report on Carcinogens
Category: chemical
Cancer Type(s): blood vessel cancer, liver, mammary gland, liver

Unraveling the Origins: Exploring 101 Triggers of Cancer

Isoprene is a naturally occurring organic compound classified as a hydrocarbon. It is produced by various plants, trees, and some microorganisms as part of their natural metabolic processes. It is one of the most abundant biogenic volatile organic compounds (BVOCs) emitted into the atmosphere. Isoprene emissions from vegetation play a significant role in the formation of atmospheric aerosols and contribute to the global carbon cycle.

1. **Industrial uses:** Isoprene is produced synthetically for various industrial applications. The largest use of synthetic isoprene is in the production of synthetic rubber, particularly in the manufacture of polyisoprene rubber, which is similar to natural rubber in its properties and applications. Isoprene rubber is used in tire manufacturing, automotive parts, conveyor belts, footwear, and other rubber products.

2. **Chemical reactivity:** Isoprene is highly reactive and readily undergoes various chemical reactions, including polymerization, oxidation, and addition reactions with other compounds. It serves as a precursor in the synthesis of various chemicals and polymers, including synthetic rubber, specialty chemicals, and pharmaceutical intermediates.

3. **Environmental impact:** Isoprene emissions from vegetation contribute to the formation of atmospheric aerosols, ozone, and secondary organic aerosols through reactions with atmospheric oxidants and other volatile organic compounds (VOCs). These aerosols have implications for air quality, climate, and human health. Isoprene emissions from industrial sources may also contribute to air pollution in urban areas.

Overall, isoprene is a versatile compound with important roles in both natural and industrial processes. Its abundance in the environment and its reactivity make it a significant player in atmospheric chemistry, climate regulation, and the global carbon cycle, while its industrial applications contribute to the production of essential materials like synthetic rubber.

According to the NTP, isoprene is listed as "reasonably anticipated to be a human carcinogen" based on sufficient evidence of carcinogenicity from studies in experimental animals, particularly mice and rats. These studies have shown increased incidences of certain types of tumors, including lung tumors, in animals exposed to isoprene through inhalation.

Trigger 64/101 – Kaposi's Sarcoma Herpesvirus

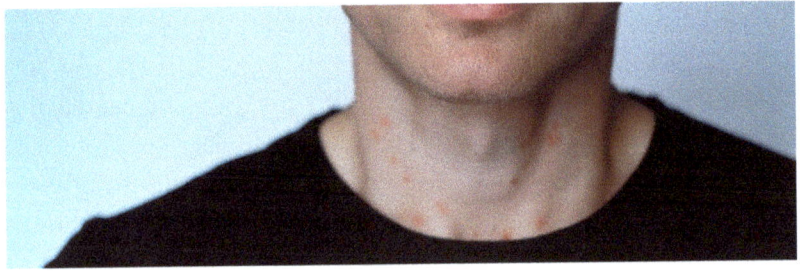

Report: 9th Report on Carcinogens
Category: biological
Cancer Type(s): skin, mouth, lymph nodes

Kaposi's sarcoma herpesvirus (KSHV), also known as human herpesvirus 8 (HHV-8), is a virus belonging to the Herpesviridae family. It is the infectious agent responsible for Kaposi's sarcoma (KS), a type of cancer that primarily affects the skin but can also involve other organs such as the mouth, lymph nodes, and internal organs.

Here are some key points about Kaposi's sarcoma herpesvirus:

Unraveling the Origins: Exploring 101 Triggers of Cancer

1. **Transmission:** KSHV is transmitted primarily through intimate contact with infected individuals. It can be spread through saliva, sexual contact, blood transfusions, and organ transplants. KSHV infection is more common in certain populations, including men who have sex with men (MSM), individuals with weakened immune systems (such as those with HIV/AIDS), and individuals from regions where KS is endemic, such as parts of Africa.

2. **Disease association:** KSHV infection is associated with several diseases, the most notable of which is Kaposi's sarcoma. KS typically presents as skin lesions, which may be red, purple, or brown in color and can vary in size and number. In addition to classic KS, which primarily affects older individuals of Mediterranean or Eastern European descent, there are several other forms of KS, including epidemic or AIDS-related KS, which occurs in individuals with HIV/AIDS, and endemic or African KS, which occurs primarily in sub-Saharan Africa.

3. **Pathogenesis:** The exact mechanisms by which KSHV causes Kaposi's sarcoma are not fully understood, but the virus is known to encode several proteins that contribute to the development and progression of the disease. These include viral oncogenes that can stimulate cell proliferation and angiogenesis (the formation of new blood vessels), as well as proteins that can inhibit the host immune response and promote tumor growth.

Overall, the oncogenic properties of Kaposi's sarcoma herpesvirus contribute to its classification as a carcinogen. Infection with KSHV increases the risk of developing Kaposi's sarcoma, particularly in individuals with weakened immune systems, such as those with HIV/AIDS or other immunocompromising conditions. Understanding the mechanisms by which KSHV promotes cancer development is essential for developing effective prevention and treatment strategies for Kaposi's sarcoma and other KSHV-associated malignancies.

Trigger 65/101 – Leather Dust

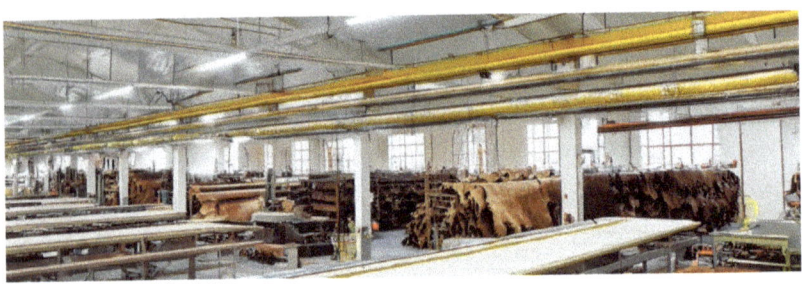

Report: ICARE study group PMID: 30922305
Category: chemical
Cancer Type(s): head, neck

Leather dust refers to the fine particles and fibers generated during the processing and manufacturing of leather products. It is produced primarily in facilities such as tanneries, leather goods manufacturing plants, and leather product finishing operations.

Here are some key points about leather dust:

1. **Generation:** Leather dust is produced during various stages of leather production, including tanning, dyeing, cutting, sewing, and finishing. It is generated when leather hides or skins are processed, treated with chemicals, cut into shape, and manipulated to create finished leather products such as shoes, bags, garments, upholstery, and accessories.

2. **Composition:** Leather dust consists of small particles and fibers derived from the processing of animal hides or skins. It may contain a variety of substances, including residual

chemicals used in the tanning and finishing processes (such as chromium salts, dyes, and preservatives), as well as organic and inorganic particulate matter from the hides themselves and from other materials used in leather manufacturing.

3. **Health hazards:** Exposure to leather dust can pose health risks to workers in the leather industry, particularly those involved in processes that generate high levels of dust, such as cutting, grinding, sanding, and buffing. Inhalation of leather dust particles can irritate the respiratory tract and may cause or exacerbate respiratory conditions such as asthma, bronchitis, and chronic obstructive pulmonary disease (COPD). Prolonged or excessive exposure to leather dust has also been associated with an increased risk of developing occupational lung diseases, including leather dust-induced lung fibrosis and occupational asthma.

4. **Prevention and control:** To minimize the health risks associated with leather dust exposure, employers in the leather industry are encouraged to implement effective dust control measures and engineering controls, such as local exhaust ventilation systems, dust collection systems, and wet suppression techniques. Personal protective equipment (PPE), such as respiratory protection (e.g., dust masks or respirators) and protective clothing, should also be provided to workers to reduce inhalation and dermal exposure to leather dust particles.

5. **Regulatory compliance:** Occupational exposure to leather dust is regulated by occupational health and safety agencies in many countries, which have established exposure limits and guidelines to protect workers from the health hazards associated with dust exposure. Employers are responsible for ensuring compliance with relevant regulations and standards

and for providing a safe working environment for their employees.

Overall, while leather dust is an inevitable byproduct of leather production, efforts to minimize dust generation and control exposure are essential to protect the health and safety of workers in the leather industry. Employers, workers, and regulatory authorities play important roles in implementing effective measures to mitigate the risks associated with leather dust exposure.

Exposure to certain components found in leather dust, such as chromium salts and other chemicals used in the tanning and finishing processes, may pose carcinogenic risks to workers in the leather industry.

Trigger 66/101 – Melphalan

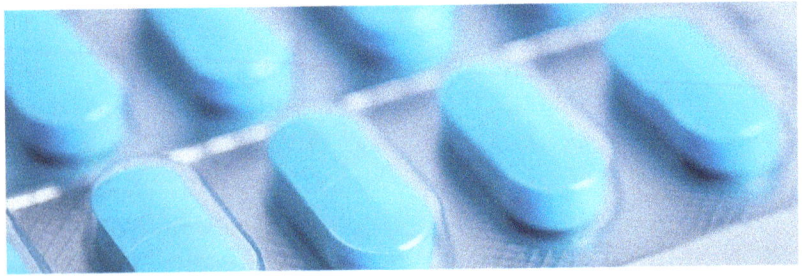

Report: 1st Report on Carcinogens
Category: chemical
Cancer Type(s): lymphatic tissue, lung, stomach

Melphalan is a chemotherapy medication belonging to the class of alkylating agents. It is primarily used in the treatment of certain types of cancer, including multiple myeloma, ovarian cancer, and melanoma. Melphalan works by interfering with the DNA replication process in rapidly dividing cancer cells, ultimately leading to cell death.

Melphalan is used as a component of combination chemotherapy regimens for the treatment of various cancers, including multiple myeloma (a type of blood cancer affecting plasma cells), ovarian cancer, and melanoma (a type of skin cancer). It may be administered orally or intravenously, depending on the specific treatment protocol and patient's condition.

Its use as a chemotherapy medication may be associated with an increased risk of secondary malignancies in some patients due to its cytotoxic and mutagenic effects on healthy cells.

Inclusion in the Report on Carcinogens does not necessarily mean that a substance is a carcinogen in all circumstances or that it directly causes cancer. Instead, it indicates that there is evidence suggesting a potential association between the substance and cancer, which may warrant further investigation or precautions in certain settings.

The classification of substances as carcinogens is based on a comprehensive evaluation of available scientific evidence by regulatory agencies and expert panels. If melphalan is included in the Report on Carcinogens, it reflects the findings of such evaluations and serves as a resource for researchers, healthcare providers, and policymakers to better understand potential health risks associated with exposure to the substance.

Trigger 67/101 – 4,4'-Methylenebis(2-chloroaniline)

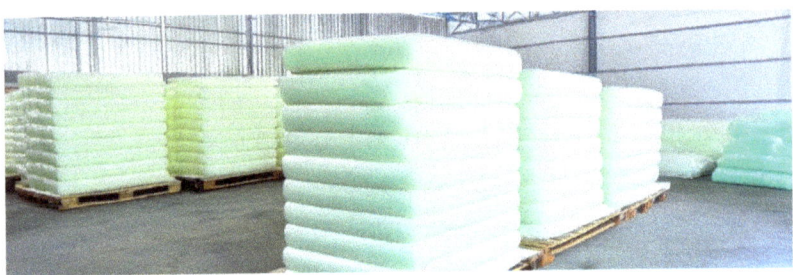

Report: National Cancer Institute CARCINOGENESIS TRS 186
Category: chemical
Cancer Type(s): bladder, thyroid

4,4'-Methylenebis(2-chloroaniline), often abbreviated as MBOCA, is a chemical compound used primarily as a curing agent in the production of polyurethane elastomers and coatings.

Here are some key points about 4,4'-Methylenebis(2-chloroaniline):

1. **Applications:** MBOCA is primarily used as a curing agent or crosslinking agent in the production of polyurethane elastomers, coatings, and adhesives. It reacts with isocyanate groups in polyurethane prepolymers to form urea linkages, thereby crosslinking the polymer chains and imparting desirable mechanical properties, such as flexibility, toughness, and abrasion resistance.

2. **Industrial usage:** MBOCA is commonly used in industries such as automotive, aerospace, construction, and manufacturing, where polyurethane materials are utilized for various applications, including seals, gaskets, rollers, conveyor belts, and molded parts.

3. **Health and safety concerns:** Exposure to MBOCA can pose health risks to workers involved in its manufacturing, handling, and processing. MBOCA is classified as a potential human carcinogen by various regulatory agencies and health organizations due to its carcinogenic properties observed in animal studies. Chronic exposure to MBOCA has been associated with an increased risk of bladder cancer and other adverse health effects, such as skin sensitization, respiratory irritation, and organ toxicity.

4. **Regulatory considerations:** Due to its carcinogenicity and health hazards, the use of MBOCA is subject to strict regulations and safety measures in many countries. Occupational exposure limits and guidelines have been established to protect workers from the risks associated with MBOCA exposure. Employers are required to implement control measures, such as engineering controls, personal protective equipment (PPE), and workplace monitoring, to minimize exposure and ensure worker safety.

4,4'-Methylenebis(2-chloroaniline) (MBOCA) is classified as a potential human carcinogen based on evidence from animal studies and limited human data. The carcinogenicity of MBOCA is primarily attributed to its ability to induce tumors, particularly bladder tumors, in laboratory animals exposed to the compound.

Animal studies have shown that chronic exposure to MBOCA can lead to the development of tumors, especially in the bladder. MBOCA is metabolized in the body to form reactive intermediates that can bind to DNA, leading to genetic mutations and cellular damage. These mutations can disrupt normal cellular processes, promote uncontrolled cell growth, and ultimately contribute to the formation of tumors.

Trigger 68/101 – 2,4,6-Trichlorophenol (TCP)

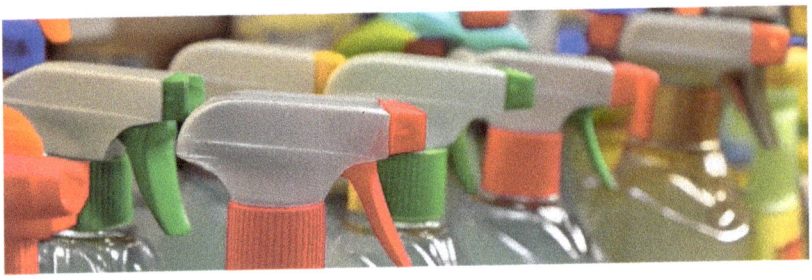

Report: 3rd Report on Carcinogens
Category: chemical
Cancer Type(s): liver, leukemia

2,4,6-Trichlorophenol (TCP) has been used for various industrial purposes, including as a biocide, fungicide, and wood preservative. It has been employed in the production of pesticides, herbicides, and disinfectants, as well as in the synthesis of other organic compounds. TCP has also been used as an intermediate in the manufacture of dyes, pharmaceuticals, and chemical intermediates.

Below are some known facts about TCP.

1. **Biocidal properties:** TCP exhibits antimicrobial properties and has been used as a biocide to control the growth of bacteria, fungi, and algae in industrial processes, water treatment systems, and wood preservation treatments. It acts by

disrupting cellular membranes and metabolic processes in microorganisms, leading to their inhibition or death.

2. **Environmental concerns:** TCP is considered a persistent organic pollutant (POP) and may persist in the environment for long periods due to its low solubility in water and resistance to degradation by microbial and chemical processes. It can bioaccumulate in living organisms and biomagnify through food chains, posing risks to aquatic organisms and wildlife. TCP contamination of soil, water, and air can occur through industrial discharges, waste disposal practices, and agricultural runoff.

3. **Health effects:** TCP exposure can have adverse health effects on humans and animals. Acute exposure to high levels of TCP vapor or dust may cause irritation of the eyes, skin, and respiratory tract. Chronic exposure to TCP through ingestion, inhalation, or dermal contact has been associated with toxic effects on the liver, kidneys, nervous system, and immune system. TCP has also been classified as a possible human carcinogen based on limited evidence from animal studies.

Due to its toxicity and environmental persistence, TCP use has been restricted or banned in some countries, and regulatory agencies have established guidelines and regulations to limit TCP emissions and protect human health and the environment. Efforts to reduce TCP contamination and exposure focus on the implementation of pollution prevention measures, waste management practices, and safer alternatives in industrial processes.

Trigger 69/101 – Nitrogen Mustard

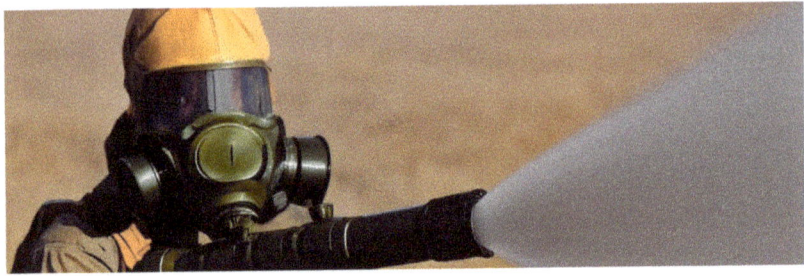

Report: 4th Report on Carcinogens
Category: chemical
Cancer Type(s): lung, thymic lymphoma

Nitrogen mustard, also known as mechlorethamine, was designed as a military agent but was later used in cancer treatment. It's one of the earliest chemotherapy agents developed and used in the treatment of cancer. While its use has decreased over time due to the development of newer and more effective chemotherapy drugs, nitrogen mustard is still occasionally used in certain medical settings for the treatment of specific types of cancer.

Mechlorethamine is primarily used in the treatment of certain types of lymphomas, such as Hodgkin lymphoma and non-Hodgkin lymphoma, as well as certain types of leukemia. It may also be used as part of combination chemotherapy regimens for other malignancies.

However, the use of mechlorethamine is limited due to its toxicity and side effects, which can include bone marrow suppression (leading to anemia, thrombocytopenia, and neutropenia), gastrointestinal symptoms, hair loss (alopecia), and increased susceptibility to infections. Additionally, mechlorethamine can cause severe skin reactions if it comes into contact with the skin.

Unraveling the Origins: Exploring 101 Triggers of Cancer

Despite its limitations, mechlorethamine remains an important treatment option for some patients with certain types of cancer, particularly those who have failed to respond to other chemotherapy drugs or who have limited treatment options available. Its use is carefully considered by oncologists and healthcare providers based on factors such as the type and stage of cancer, the patient's overall health status, and treatment goals.

Overall, while the use of nitrogen mustard has declined over time, it continues to have a role in cancer treatment in certain situations, particularly in the management of lymphomas and leukemias. Research into new treatment modalities and targeted therapies continues to advance, providing additional options for patients with cancer.

Trigger 70/101 – Antimony Trioxide

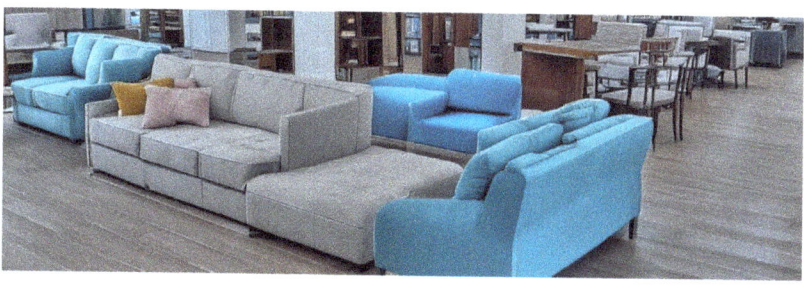

Report: National Toxicology Program TR 590
Category: chemical
Cancer Type(s): lung

Antimony trioxide has several industrial applications, primarily as a flame-retardant synergist and as a catalyst in the production of polyethylene terephthalate (PET) plastics. It is commonly used as a flame-retardant additive in plastics, textiles, rubber, and other materials to reduce the flammability of products and enhance fire safety. Antimony trioxide acts as a flame-retardant synergist by promoting the formation of a protective char layer that inhibits combustion.

Antimony trioxide functions as a flame retardant by releasing antimony oxide radicals (Sb_2O_5) when exposed to heat or flames. These radicals act as free radical scavengers, interrupting the combustion chain reaction and reducing the rate of flame spread. Additionally, antimony trioxide can form a glassy, protective layer on the surface of materials, which helps to prevent the ignition and propagation of flames.

While antimony trioxide is effective as a flame retardant, there are concerns about its potential health and environmental impacts. Prolonged exposure to antimony trioxide dust or fumes may cause respiratory irritation, skin irritation, and eye irritation. In addition, antimony trioxide is classified as a possible human carcinogen by some regulatory agencies based on animal studies showing an increased incidence of lung tumors in rats exposed to high doses of antimony trioxide.

Overall, antimony trioxide is an important flame-retardant additive used in various industries to improve the fire safety of materials and products. However, precautions should be taken to minimize exposure to antimony trioxide dust or fumes and to mitigate potential health and environmental risks associated with its use.

Antimony trioxide has been shown to exhibit genotoxic effects in some in vitro and in vivo studies. Genotoxicity refers to the ability of a substance to cause damage to the genetic material (DNA) of cells, leading to mutations that can contribute to the initiation and progression of cancer. While the mechanisms by which antimony trioxide induces genotoxicity are not fully understood, it

Unraveling the Origins: Exploring 101 Triggers of Cancer

is thought to involve the formation of reactive oxygen species (ROS) and DNA damage.

Trigger 71/101 – Arsenic

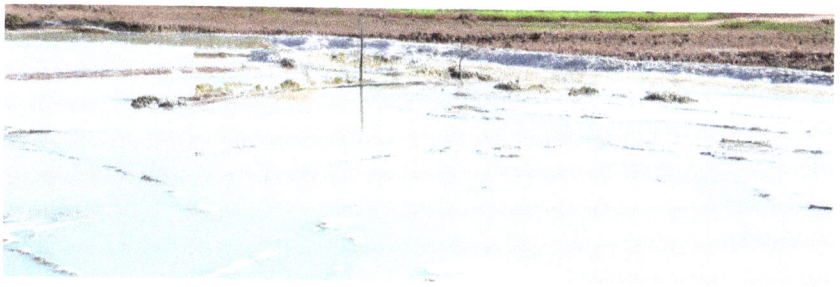

Report: 1st Report on Carcinogens
Carcinogen Category: chemical
Cancer Type(s): skin, lung, digestive tract, liver, bladder, kidney, lymphatic

Arsenic and its compounds have been used for various purposes throughout history, including in agriculture, industry, and medicine. However, arsenic is also highly toxic to humans and other organisms. Ingesting or inhaling high levels of arsenic can cause acute poisoning, while long-term exposure to lower levels can lead to chronic arsenic poisoning, which is associated with a range of health problems including skin lesions, cancer, cardiovascular diseases, and neurological effects.

Extraction and processing of metal ores can release arsenic into the environment. Arsenic contamination of groundwater is a significant concern in many parts of the world, particularly in regions where groundwater is the primary source of drinking water. Contamination can occur naturally or as a result of human activities such as mining, industrial processes, and the use of arsenic-containing pesticides.

Arsenic can be found in various products and substances, both naturally and as a result of human activities. Some common sources of arsenic include:

1. **Drinking water**: Arsenic contamination of groundwater is a significant concern in many parts of the world, particularly in regions where groundwater is the primary source of drinking water.

2. **Food**: Arsenic can be present in certain foods, particularly in rice and seafood. Rice tends to accumulate arsenic from water and soil, while seafood can contain organic forms of arsenic as well as inorganic arsenic from environmental sources.

3. **Wood preservatives**: Arsenic was historically used in wood preservatives, particularly in pressure-treated lumber used in outdoor structures like decks, playground equipment, and fences. However, the use of arsenic-based wood preservatives has been largely phased out in many countries due to health concerns.

4. **Pesticides**: Arsenic-based pesticides were once commonly used in agriculture, particularly in the past for controlling pests in cotton fields, orchards, and vineyards. While their use has declined significantly, residues of arsenic-based pesticides may still be present in soil in some areas.

5. **Industrial processes**: Arsenic may be released into the environment as a byproduct of various industrial processes, including mining, smelting, and coal combustion. Workers in industries such as metal smelting and electronics manufacturing may be at risk of exposure to arsenic.

6. **Consumer products**: Arsenic may be present in certain consumer products, such as some types of cosmetics, herbal

Unraveling the Origins: Exploring 101 Triggers of Cancer

remedies, and dietary supplements. Regulatory agencies monitor these products for arsenic content to ensure consumer safety.

It's important to note that exposure to high levels of arsenic can pose serious health risks, including acute poisoning and long-term health effects such as cancer and cardiovascular disease. Efforts to monitor and regulate arsenic levels in various products and the environment are important for protecting public health.

Trigger 72/101 – Untreated Mineral Oils

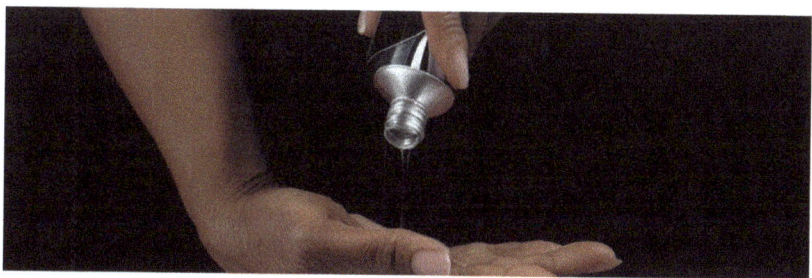

Report: 1st Report on Carcinogens
Category: chemical
Cancer Type(s): skin

Untreated mineral oils are petroleum-based oils that have undergone minimal processing or refinement and are used in various industrial and commercial applications. Here are some key points about untreated mineral oils:

1. **Composition:** Untreated mineral oils are derived from crude oil through distillation and refining processes. They consist mainly of hydrocarbons, including alkanes, cycloalkanes, and aromatic compounds, with varying molecular weights and

chemical compositions depending on the source of the crude oil and the refining process used.

2. **Properties:** Untreated mineral oils typically have a clear or pale yellow appearance and a relatively low viscosity, making them suitable for use as lubricants, hydraulic fluids, cutting oils, and insulating fluids. They have good thermal stability, chemical inertness, and low volatility, which make them useful in applications where temperature extremes, chemical exposure, and oxidation resistance are important.

3. **Applications:** Untreated mineral oils have a wide range of industrial and commercial applications due to their lubricating, insulating, and protective properties. They are commonly used as lubricants in machinery and equipment, hydraulic fluids in hydraulic systems, cutting oils in metalworking processes, and insulating fluids in electrical transformers and capacitors. Untreated mineral oils may also be used as carrier oils in cosmetics, pharmaceuticals, and personal care products.

4. **Health and Environmental Considerations:** While untreated mineral oils are generally considered safe for their intended applications, there may be concerns about potential health and environmental risks associated with prolonged or excessive exposure. Mineral oils may contain trace amounts of impurities, such as polycyclic aromatic hydrocarbons (PAHs), which are known to be carcinogenic. Additionally, spills or leaks of untreated mineral oils can contaminate soil, water, and air, leading to environmental pollution and adverse effects on ecosystems.

Overall, untreated mineral oils are versatile and widely used industrial chemicals that play a crucial role in many industrial processes and applications. However, proper handling, storage, and disposal practices are important to minimize potential risks to human health and the environment associated with their use

Untreated mineral oils are used in a variety of personal care products due to their emollient and moisturizing properties. Here are some examples of personal care products that may contain untreated mineral oils:

1. **Moisturizers and Lotions:** Untreated mineral oils are commonly used in moisturizing creams, lotions, and body oils to hydrate and soften the skin. They help to form a protective barrier on the skin's surface, preventing moisture loss and improving skin texture.

2. **Lip Balms and Lipsticks:** Untreated mineral oils are often included in lip balms, lipsticks, and lip glosses to provide hydration and shine to the lips. They help to moisturize dry and chapped lips, keeping them soft and supple.

3. **Baby Care Products:** Untreated mineral oils are found in many baby care products, such as baby oils, lotions, and diaper creams. They are gentle and soothing on delicate baby skin, helping to prevent dryness and irritation.

4. **Hair Care Products:** Untreated mineral oils may be used in hair care products, such as shampoos, conditioners, and hair oils, to condition and nourish the hair and scalp. They help to smooth and soften the hair, reduce frizz, and improve manageability.

5. **Makeup Removers:** Untreated mineral oils are commonly used as ingredients in makeup removers and cleansing oils. They help to dissolve and remove makeup, dirt, and impurities from the skin's surface without stripping away natural oils.

6. **Sunscreen Products:** Untreated mineral oils are sometimes included in sunscreen formulations as emollients and moisturizers. They help to keep the skin hydrated and prevent dryness, particularly in sunscreens with high SPF values that can be drying to the skin.

7. **Shaving Creams and Lotions:** Untreated mineral oils are used in some shaving creams and lotions to provide lubrication and glide for a smooth and comfortable shave. They help to soften the hair and moisturize the skin, reducing irritation and razor burn.

It's always a good idea to check the ingredient list and perform a patch test before using new products, especially if you have sensitive skin or allergies.

Trigger 73/101 – Nickel Compounds

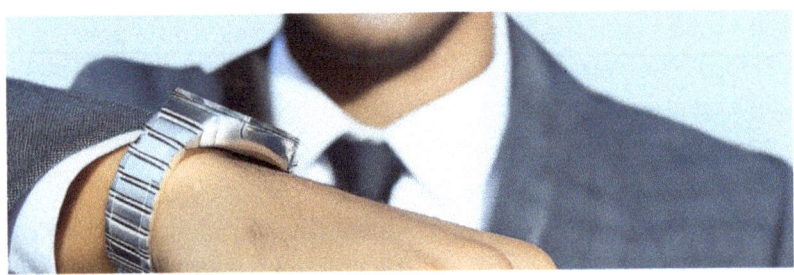

Report: 10th Report on Carcinogens
Category: environment
Cancer Type(s): lung, nasal

Nickel compounds are chemical compounds that contain the element nickel in combination with other elements. Nickel compounds can vary widely in their chemical and physical properties depending on the specific elements they are combined with and the chemical bonds present.

Nickel compounds have a wide range of industrial applications due to their various properties. Nickel oxide is commonly used as a catalyst in chemical reactions, as a pigment in ceramics and glass, and in the production of batteries. Nickel sulfate is used in electroplating processes to deposit nickel onto metal surfaces. Nickel chloride is used in the production of nickel-cadmium batteries and as a catalyst in organic synthesis.

Some nickel compounds can be toxic to humans and the environment. Nickel and certain nickel compounds have been classified as human carcinogens by regulatory agencies such as the International Agency for Research on Cancer (IARC) and the U.S. Environmental Protection Agency (EPA). Inhalation or ingestion of nickel compounds, as well as dermal contact, can lead to adverse health effects, including respiratory irritation, skin sensitization, allergic reactions, and lung cancer.

In addition to their carcinogenic effects, nickel compounds can also cause other adverse health effects, including respiratory irritation, skin sensitization, allergic reactions, and lung damage. Regulatory agencies such as the U.S. Environmental Protection Agency (EPA) have established regulations and guidelines to limit exposure to nickel compounds in occupational and environmental settings to protect human health. Efforts to minimize exposure to nickel compounds include the use of engineering controls, personal protective equipment (PPE), and workplace monitoring to reduce occupational exposure, as well as pollution prevention measures to minimize environmental releases of nickel compounds.

Some watches may contain nickel compounds, particularly in components such as watch cases, buckles, clasps, and metal watch bands. Nickel is commonly used in the production of stainless steel, which is a popular material for watchmaking due to its durability, corrosion resistance, and aesthetic appeal. Stainless steel typically contains nickel as one of its alloying elements, along with iron, chromium, and other metals.

While stainless steel is generally considered safe for most people, nickel allergy is a common concern, as nickel is one of the most common causes of allergic contact dermatitis (nickel dermatitis). Individuals who are allergic or sensitive to nickel may experience skin irritation, redness, itching, or rash when their skin comes into contact with nickel-containing materials, such as stainless steel.

To address concerns about nickel allergy, some watch manufacturers may use hypoallergenic materials or coatings to reduce nickel exposure in their products. For example, watches with a stainless steel caseback may have a protective coating or barrier to prevent direct skin contact with nickel. Additionally, certain watch bands may be made from alternative materials that are less likely to cause allergic reactions, such as leather, silicone, rubber, or fabric.

If you have a known nickel allergy or sensitivity, it's important to choose watches and watch bands that are labeled as hypoallergenic or nickel-free to minimize the risk of skin irritation or allergic reactions. Additionally, keeping the skin dry and clean, avoiding prolonged contact with nickel-containing materials, and using protective barriers such as clear nail polish or barrier creams can help reduce the risk of nickel dermatitis for individuals with nickel allergy.

Unraveling the Origins: Exploring 101 Triggers of Cancer

Trigger 74/101 – Amitrole

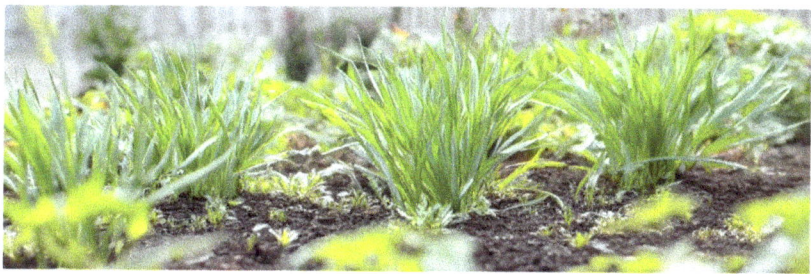

Report: 2nd Report on Carcinogens
Category: chemical
Cancer Type(s): thyroid, pituitary, liver

Amitrole, also known as aminotriazole, is a non-selective herbicide that has been used in agriculture for weed control. However, its use has been restricted or banned in many countries due to concerns about its potential health and environmental risks.

In the past, amitrole was widely used to control weeds in various crops, including cereals, fruits, vegetables, and ornamental plants. It was effective against a broad spectrum of weeds and was commonly applied as a pre-planting or pre-emergence herbicide to prevent weed growth in agricultural fields.

However, concerns about the safety of amitrole have led to restrictions on its use in many parts of the world. The European Union, for example, has banned the use of amitrole as an herbicide since 2002 due to its classification as a suspected human carcinogen and its potential to contaminate groundwater.

In the United States, amitrole is classified as a restricted-use pesticide, meaning it can only be applied by certified applicators and is subject to strict regulations and usage restrictions. The U.S.

Environmental Protection Agency (EPA) has also imposed limitations on the use of amitrole to reduce potential risks to human health and the environment.

The classification of amitrole as a potential carcinogen is primarily based on studies conducted in laboratory animals, particularly rodents, which have shown that exposure to amitrole can increase the incidence of tumors in various organs. Here are some key points regarding the carcinogenicity of amitrole:

Studies in animals, particularly rats and mice, have demonstrated that exposure to amitrole is associated with an increased incidence of tumors, particularly thyroid tumors and liver tumors. These studies typically involve administering high doses of amitrole to animals over extended periods and observing the development of tumors over time.

In addition to thyroid tumors, some animal studies have also reported an increased incidence of liver tumors in rats and mice exposed to amitrole. Liver tumors observed in these studies include hepatocellular adenomas and carcinomas, which are considered malignant tumors.

Amitrole has been shown to cause DNA damage and mutations in laboratory studies, suggesting a potential genotoxic effect. Additionally, amitrole may disrupt thyroid hormone homeostasis and thyroid function, leading to thyroid gland hyperplasia and tumor formation.

Unraveling the Origins: Exploring 101 Triggers of Cancer

Trigger 75/101 – Basic Red 9 Monohydrochloride

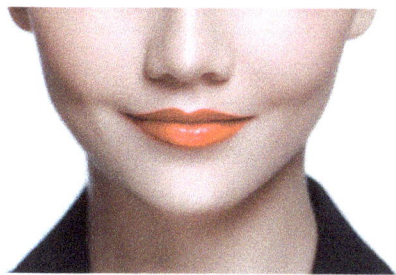

Report: 5th Report on Carcinogens
Category: chemical
Cancer Type(s): bladder, liver

Basic Red 9 Monohydrochloride, also known as Crystal Scarlet, is a synthetic dye belonging to the family of cationic dyes. It is commonly used as a colorant in various industries, including textiles, cosmetics, and food.

Here are some key points about Basic Red 9 Monohydrochloride:

Basic Red 9 Monohydrochloride typically appears as a dark red or maroon powder or granules. It is soluble in water, producing a red-colored solution.

Basic Red 9 Monohydrochloride is primarily used as a colorant or dye in various applications. In the textile industry, it is used to dye natural and synthetic fibers, such as cotton, wool, silk, and polyester, to impart a vibrant red or pink color. In the cosmetics industry, it may be used in hair dyes, shampoos, soaps, and other personal care products to add color. Additionally, Basic Red 9 Monohydrochloride may be used as a colorant in food products, although its use in food is subject to regulatory approval and restrictions in some countries.

The concern about the carcinogenicity of certain synthetic dyes arises from the presence of aromatic amines, which can be formed as impurities during the manufacturing process or through metabolic breakdown in the body. Some aromatic amines have been shown to have carcinogenic properties in animal studies and are classified as potential human carcinogens.

It's important to note that the carcinogenicity of synthetic dyes, including Basic Red 9 Monohydrochloride, depends on factors such as the specific chemical composition, purity, and usage patterns. Proper regulatory oversight, adherence to safety guidelines, and ongoing research are essential for ensuring the safe use of synthetic dyes in various applications while minimizing potential health risks to consumers and workers.

Trigger 76/101 – Acetaldehyde

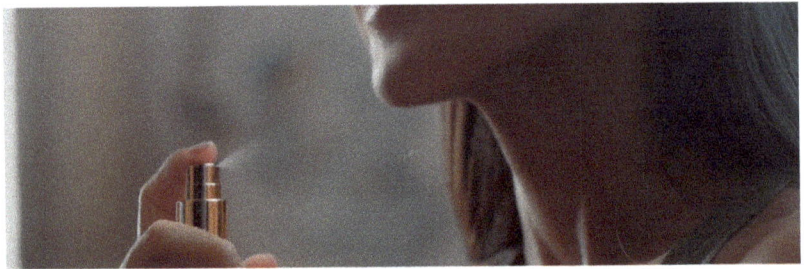

Report: 6th Report on Carcinogens
Category: chemical
Cancer Type(s): nasal, bone, mammary

Acetaldehyde is an organic chemical compound that is part of the aldehyde group. Industrially, acetaldehyde is produced mainly by the oxidation of ethanol or by the hydration of acetylene.

Unraveling the Origins: Exploring 101 Triggers of Cancer

Applications include:

1. Chemical Industry: Used as an intermediate in the synthesis of acetic acid, peracetic acid, pentaerythritol, and other chemicals.
2. Pharmaceuticals: Involved in the production of various drugs.
3. Perfumes and Flavors: Utilized for its pleasant fruity scent in perfumes and as a flavoring agent.
4. Plastics and Resins: Used in the manufacture of certain plastics and synthetic resins.
5. Disinfectants and Preservatives: Employed due to its antimicrobial properties.
6. Rubber Industry: Utilized in the vulcanization process of rubber.
7. Agricultural Chemicals: An intermediate in the production of pesticides and herbicides.

Despite its widespread use, acetaldehyde is also recognized as a potentially harmful substance. It is classified as a probable human carcinogen, and exposure to high levels can cause health issues. Therefore, its handling and usage are regulated in many countries to ensure safety.

Trigger 77/101 – 1-Bromopropane

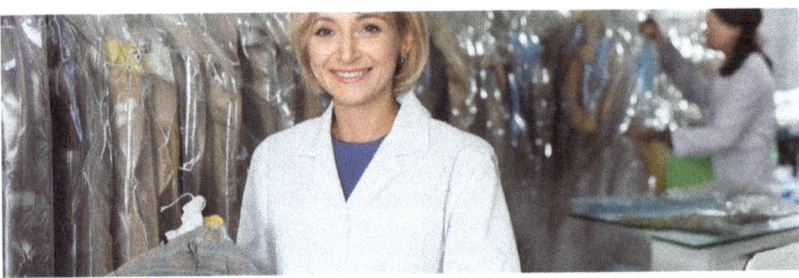

Report: 13th Report on Carcinogens
Category: chemical
Cancer Type(s): skin, colon

1-Bromopropane, also known as n-propyl bromide or nPB, is an organic compound that belongs to the class of alkyl bromides. Widely used as a solvent in industrial and commercial applications, including degreasing, cleaning of metals and electronics, and dry cleaning.

1. Chemical Intermediate: Used in the synthesis of pharmaceuticals, agrochemicals, and other organic compounds.
2. **Adhesives and Sealants**: Utilized in the production of adhesives, sealants, and coatings.

1-Bromopropane is known to be toxic, and exposure can affect the central nervous system, reproductive system, and respiratory system. It can cause headaches, dizziness, nausea, and, in severe cases, neurotoxicity. Being volatile, it can contribute to air pollution and has implications for both environmental health and worker safety. 1-Bromopropane has been identified as a potential ozone-depleting substance, though its impact is less significant compared to other brominated compounds.

Bromopropane (nPB) is considered a carcinogen due to its ability to cause changes in cellular structures and functions that can lead to cancer. Occupational exposure studies have shown an increased incidence of certain cancers among workers who are regularly exposed to 1-bromopropane. This epidemiological data supports the classification of 1-bromopropane as a potential carcinogen.

Trigger 78/101 – Chloramphenicol

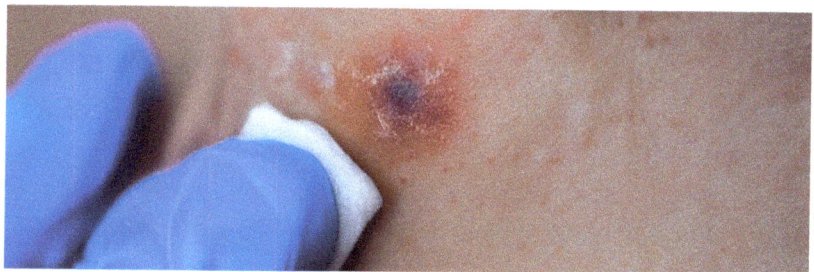

Report: 10th Report on Carcinogens
Category: chemical
Cancer Type(s): leukemia

Chloramphenicol is a broad-spectrum antibiotic that is used to treat a variety of bacterial infections. It was first isolated from the bacterium *Streptomyces venezuelae* in 1947 and was the first antibiotic to be manufactured synthetically on a large scale.

Chloramphenicol works by inhibiting bacterial protein synthesis. It binds to the 50S subunit of the bacterial ribosome, preventing the peptide bond formation necessary for protein synthesis. This action is generally bacteriostatic, meaning it inhibits the growth and reproduction of bacteria. It is effective against a wide range of Gram-positive and Gram-negative bacteria, as well as some anaerobic organisms. Commonly used to treat infections such as meningitis, typhoid fever, and certain types of respiratory and eye infections.

One of the most serious side effects of chloramphenicol is its potential to cause bone marrow suppression, which can lead to aplastic anemia, a potentially fatal condition. This risk has significantly limited its use. In neonates, chloramphenicol can cause a condition known as gray baby syndrome, characterized by vomiting, abdominal distension, cyanosis, and, in severe cases, death. This occurs because infants' livers cannot metabolize the drug effectively.

In summary, chloramphenicol is a potent antibiotic with a broad spectrum of activity but is associated with significant risks, particularly bone marrow suppression and gray baby syndrome. Its use is typically reserved for severe infections where other antibiotics are not suitable.

The primary concern associated with chloramphenicol is its potential to cause bone marrow suppression and aplastic anemia, particularly with prolonged or high-dose use.
In addition to bone marrow suppression, chloramphenicol can cause other adverse effects, including gray baby syndrome in newborns and hypersensitivity reactions.

Unraveling the Origins: Exploring 101 Triggers of Cancer

Trigger 79/101 – Dacarbazine

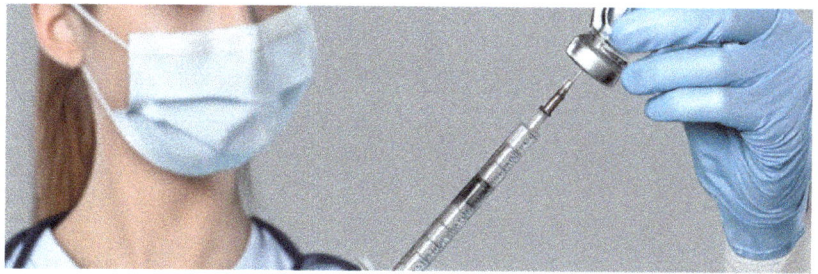

Report: 4th Report on Carcinogens
Category: chemical
Cancer Type(s): non-lymphoblastic leukemia

Dacarbazine, also known by its trade name DTIC-Dome, is a chemotherapy medication used to treat various types of cancer. Dacarbazine is a synthetic derivative of triazine and belongs to the class of alkylating agents.

Dacarbazine works by interfering with the DNA synthesis and repair processes in rapidly dividing cancer cells. It forms methylated adducts with DNA, leading to DNA damage and ultimately cell death. As an alkylating agent, dacarbazine primarily targets cancer cells that are actively dividing, although it can also affect normal cells to some extent.

Dacarbazine is used to treat various types of cancer, including metastatic melanoma, Hodgkin's lymphoma, soft tissue sarcoma, and neuroblastoma. It is often used in combination with other chemotherapy drugs or as part of multidrug regimens for more effective cancer treatment.

Dacarbazine is a cytotoxic drug with potential risks to healthcare workers and patients, so proper handling and administration procedures must be followed to minimize exposure.

In summary, while it can be effective in killing cancer cells, it also carries risks of side effects and requires careful monitoring during treatment.

Trigger 80/101 – Danthron

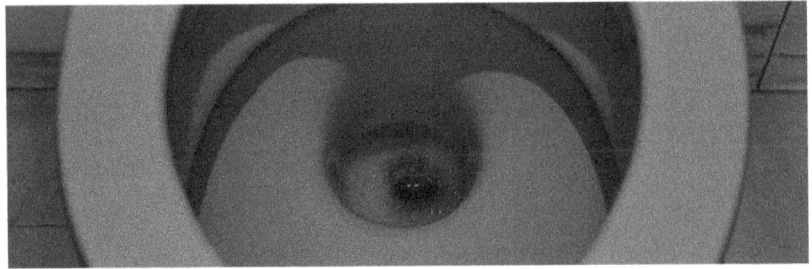

Report: 4th Report on Carcinogens
Category: chemical
Cancer Type(s): non-lymphoblastic leukemia

Danthron, also known as chrysazin or 1,8-dihydroxyanthraquinone is a naturally occurring anthraquinone derivative found in plants such as senna (Cassia species) and rhubarb (Rheum species).

Danthron has a long history of use in traditional medicine, particularly as a laxative and purgative agent. It has been used for centuries in various cultures to relieve constipation and promote bowel movements. Senna leaves, which contain danthron and related compounds, are commonly used as herbal laxatives in over-the-counter products and natural remedies.

Danthron works primarily by stimulating peristalsis, the rhythmic contraction of the intestinal muscles, which helps move stool through the colon and promote bowel movements. It acts as a laxative by increasing the secretion of water and electrolytes into the colon and softening the stool, making it easier to pass.

While danthron has been used historically as a laxative, its safety and efficacy have been called into question in recent years. The U.S. Food and Drug Administration (FDA) has issued warnings about the use of products containing danthron due to concerns about its potential side effects, including gastrointestinal irritation, electrolyte imbalances, and liver toxicity.

Due to the safety issues associated with danthron, alternative treatments for constipation, such as dietary changes, increased fluid intake, and the use of other laxatives (e.g., bulk-forming agents, osmotic laxatives), are often recommended as first-line options. Herbal remedies containing other laxative compounds, such as senna without danthron, may also be considered as alternatives for relieving constipation.

In summary, danthron is a naturally occurring compound with a history of use as a laxative and purgative agent. While it has been used traditionally for constipation relief, concerns about its safety and potential side effects have led to regulatory restrictions in some countries. Alternative treatments for constipation are available and may be preferred due to their safety profile.

Danthron has been shown to exhibit genotoxic effects in various in vitro and in vivo studies. Genotoxicity refers to the ability of a substance to cause damage to the genetic material (DNA) of cells, potentially leading to mutations and the development of cancer. Studies have demonstrated that danthron can induce DNA damage, chromosomal aberrations, and mutations in bacterial and mammalian cells exposed to the compound.

Trigger 81/101 – Furan

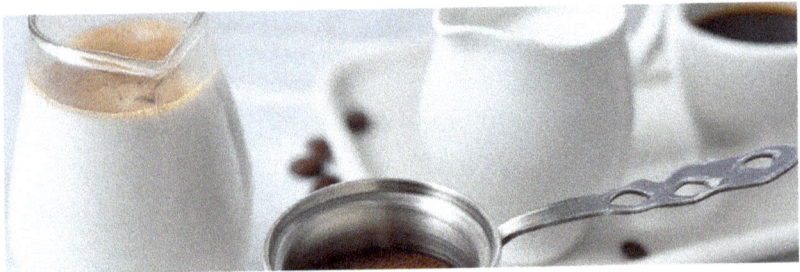

Report: 8th Report on Carcinogens
Category: chemical
Cancer Type(s): liver, adrenal, leukemia

Furan is used as a starting material in the synthesis of various chemicals, including pharmaceuticals, agrochemicals, and polymer precursors. Furan is found in trace amounts in various natural sources, including certain foods, beverages, and tobacco smoke. It is a component of the aroma and flavor of some foods, such as coffee, baked goods, and grilled meats, contributing to their characteristic smell and taste. It serves as a building block for the production of other furan derivatives, such as furfural, which is used in the manufacture of resins, solvents, and agricultural chemicals.

Furan is considered to be potentially hazardous to human health due to its toxicity and carcinogenicity. Chronic exposure to furan has been associated with adverse health effects, including liver toxicity, kidney damage, and carcinogenesis in animal studies. Occupational exposure to furan vapor or ingestion of foods contaminated with furan may pose health risks, particularly in industrial settings where furan is produced or used.

Regulatory agencies such as the U.S. Environmental Protection Agency (EPA) and the European Chemicals Agency (ECHA) have classified furan as a possible human carcinogen based on animal studies demonstrating carcinogenic effects.

Below are some examples of foods that may contain furan:

1. **Coffee**:

    - Furan can form during the roasting process of coffee beans, particularly when beans are roasted at high temperatures. Therefore, brewed coffee may contain trace levels of furan.
    - The exact furan content in coffee can vary depending on factors such as the roasting temperature, brewing method, and storage conditions.

2. **Baked Goods**:

    - Furan can be generated during the baking or heating of bread, pastries, and other baked goods, especially when baked at high temperatures.
    - Bakery products that are browned or toasted may contain slightly higher levels of furan due to the Maillard reaction, which occurs between amino acids and reducing sugars during baking.

3. **Canned Foods**:

    - Furan can form in canned foods during the sterilization process, particularly when acidic foods are canned using high-temperature methods.
    - Canned fruits, vegetables, soups, and sauces may contain trace amounts of furan, although levels are typically low and considered safe for consumption.

4. **Processed Meats**:

- Furan can be formed during the cooking or processing of certain meats, particularly when meat is grilled, broiled, or pan-fried at high temperatures.
- Processed meats such as sausages, bacon, and ham may contain small amounts of furan, although the contribution from these sources to overall dietary furan exposure is relatively low compared to other foods.

5. **Alcoholic Beverages**:

- Furan can form during the fermentation and distillation processes of alcoholic beverages, particularly spirits such as whisky, brandy, and rum.
- While furan levels in alcoholic beverages are generally low, certain production methods and aging processes may influence furan content in specific products.

It's important to note that the levels of furan in these foods are typically low.

Unraveling the Origins: Exploring 101 Triggers of Cancer

Trigger 82/101 – Methylaziridine

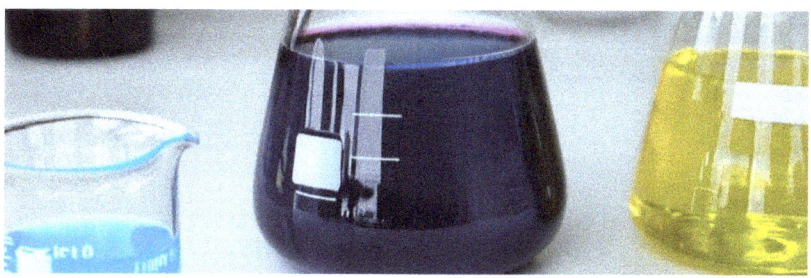

Report: 4th Report on Carcinogens
Category: chemical
Cancer Type(s): mammary leukemia

Methylaziridine, also known as 1-Methylaziridine or N-Methylaziridine is primarily used in organic synthesis and chemical research due to its reactive nature. Its applications include:

1. **Chemical Synthesis**: It serves as a building block for the synthesis of more complex molecules.

2. **Pharmaceuticals**: It may be used in the synthesis of pharmaceuticals and biologically active compounds.

3. **Polymer Chemistry**: Methylaziridine can be involved in the production of specialized polymers and materials due to its reactive aziridine ring.

Applications in Pharmaceuticals:

1. **Synthesis of Active Pharmaceutical Ingredients (APIs)**: Methylaziridine and its derivatives can be

intermediates in the synthesis of more complex molecules. These intermediates are crucial steps in the production of various APIs.

2. **Alkylating Agents**: Certain aziridines are used as alkylating agents in chemotherapy drugs. These compounds can interfere with DNA replication in cancer cells, thus inhibiting their growth. However, methylaziridine itself is not directly used due to its high toxicity and non-selectivity.

3. **Precursor for Drug Design**: The reactivity of the aziridine ring makes it useful in the design and synthesis of novel compounds with potential pharmacological activity. Researchers often modify the aziridine ring to create new molecules that can be tested for therapeutic effects.

While methylaziridine itself is not a drug, here are some related compounds that have been explored for pharmaceutical use:

1. **Mitomycin C**: A well-known chemotherapeutic agent that contains an aziridine ring. It is used to treat various cancers, including stomach and pancreatic cancer.

2. **Thiotepa**: Another chemotherapeutic agent that includes an aziridine ring in its structure. It is used in the treatment of bladder cancer and certain types of breast cancer.

3. **AZT (Zidovudine)**: An antiviral drug used in the treatment of HIV/AIDS. While AZT itself does not contain an aziridine ring, some of its synthetic routes involve aziridine intermediates.

4. its structural motif plays a significant role in the synthesis and development of various drugs. Researchers continue to explore the potential of aziridine derivatives in creating new and effective therapeutic agents.

Methylaziridine is considered a potential carcinogen primarily due to its highly reactive aziridine ring, which can interact with biological molecules, including DNA. This reactivity can lead to mutations, which are changes in the DNA sequence. If such mutations occur in critical regions of the genome, they can disrupt normal cell function and potentially lead to the development of cancer. Here are the key reasons for its carcinogenic potential:

Methylaziridine's carcinogenic potential stems from its ability to chemically interact with DNA, causing mutations and disrupting normal cellular functions. This can initiate a cascade of events leading to cancer. Therefore, strict safety measures are essential when handling this compound to minimize exposure and potential health risks.

Trigger 83/101 – Metronidazole

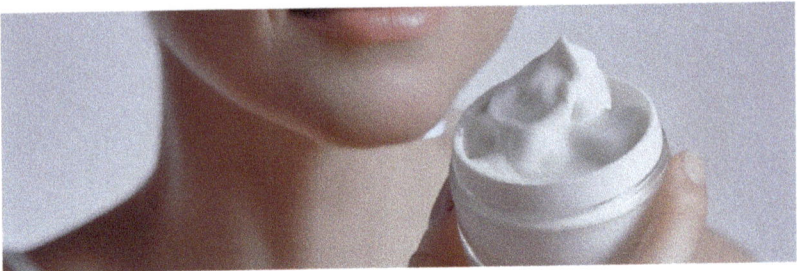

Report: 4th Report on Carcinogens
Category: chemical
Cancer Type(s): uterine cervix, lung

Metronidazole is an antibiotic and antiprotozoal medication widely used to treat a variety of infections. It belongs to the nitroimidazole class of drugs and is effective against anaerobic bacteria and certain parasites.

Metronidazole works by entering the cells of anaerobic bacteria and protozoa, where its nitro group is reduced by cellular proteins to reactive intermediates. These intermediates interact with the DNA of the microorganisms, leading to inhibition of nucleic acid synthesis and eventually causing cell death.

Metronidazole is used to treat a variety of infections, including:

1. **Bacterial Vaginosis**: Effective against Gardnerella vaginalis and other bacteria causing this condition.

2. **Amebiasis**: Used to treat infections caused by Entamoeba histolytica.

3. **Trichomoniasis**: Treats infections caused by the protozoan Trichomonas vaginalis.

4. **Giardiasis**: Effective against Giardia lamblia infections.

5. **Anaerobic Bacterial Infections**: Includes infections like intra-abdominal infections, skin infections, respiratory tract infections, and bone and joint infections.

6. **Clostridium difficile-associated Diarrhea**: Used in the treatment of C. difficile colitis.

Metronidazole is one of the most commonly prescribed antibiotics worldwide due to its effectiveness against a broad spectrum of anaerobic bacteria and certain protozoa.

Estimated Usage:

1. **Hospital Settings**: Metronidazole is frequently used in hospital settings for the treatment of serious anaerobic infections, such as intra-abdominal infections and infections associated with surgery.

2. **Outpatient Prescriptions**: Many outpatient clinics and primary care physicians prescribe metronidazole for various infections, making it one of the most commonly prescribed antibiotics in outpatient settings.

3. **Global Impact**: Metronidazole is included in the World Health Organization's List of Essential Medicines, highlighting its importance in healthcare systems worldwide.

Millions of individuals receive prescriptions for metronidazole each year. Its widespread use underscores its significance in the treatment of various infections and its impact on global public health.

Trigger 84/101 – Nitrofen

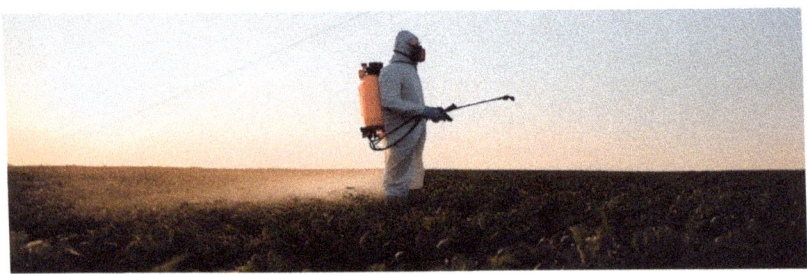

Report: 3rd Report on Carcinogens
Category: chemical
Cancer Type(s): liver, pancreas

Nitrofen, also known by its trade names as Tok, Nitrofene, and Karmex, is a synthetic herbicide belonging to the chemical class of nitrophenyl ethers. It was primarily used to control a broad spectrum of weeds in various crops, including cereals, fruits, vegetables, and ornamentals. Nitrofen works by inhibiting the photosynthetic electron transport chain in plants, leading to their death. Nitrofen can persist in the environment for an extended period, posing risks of contamination to soil, water, and non-target organisms.

Nitrofen is considered toxic to humans and animals. Acute exposure to high doses can cause irritation to the skin, eyes, and respiratory tract. Chronic exposure may lead to more severe health effects, including liver and kidney damage, as well as potential carcinogenicity. Nitrofen can leach into groundwater and surface water bodies, leading to contamination. Its persistence in soil can also pose risks to non-target plants and organisms.

Nitrofen was banned for use in the United States in 1992. The U.S. Environmental Protection Agency (EPA) revoked all registrations for nitrofen-containing products due to concerns over its potential health and environmental risks. This decision was part of the EPA's efforts to reassess the safety of pesticides and herbicides and to implement stricter regulations to protect human health and the environment.

The ban on nitrofen in the United States was prompted by evidence of its persistence in the environment, potential toxicity to humans and wildlife, and concerns about its carcinogenicity. Following the ban, the EPA prohibited the sale, distribution, and use of products containing nitrofen as an active ingredient, effectively removing it from the market.

Trigger 85/101 – Norethisterone

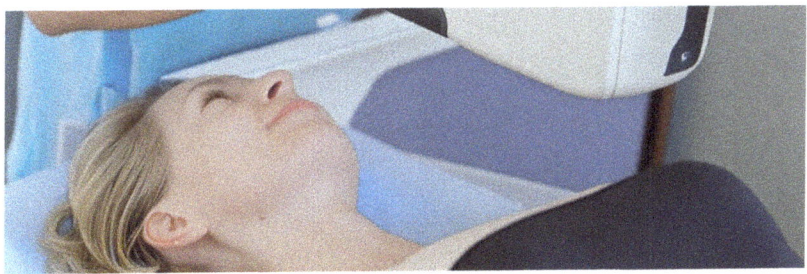

Report: 4th Report on Carcinogens
Category: chemical
Cancer Type(s): pituitary-gland, mammary

Norethisterone, also known as norethindrone, is a synthetic progestin hormone that is structurally similar to the naturally occurring hormone progesterone. It is widely used in medicine, particularly in hormonal contraceptives and hormone replacement therapy (HRT) for women. Norethisterone is also used in the treatment of various gynecological conditions and menstrual disorders. These contraceptives are used by millions of women worldwide to prevent pregnancy.

Norethisterone may be prescribed to regulate menstrual cycles, treat irregular or heavy menstrual bleeding (menorrhagia), manage conditions like endometriosis, and alleviate symptoms of premenstrual syndrome (PMS). The number of individuals using norethisterone for these indications depends on the prevalence of these conditions and individual patient needs.

Norethisterone, like other synthetic hormones used in hormonal contraceptives and hormone replacement therapy, has been studied for potential links to cancer. The classification of norethisterone and similar compounds as potential carcinogens arises from evidence suggesting that prolonged use of hormonal treatments can increase the risk of certain types of cancer.

Here are some key points regarding the potential carcinogenicity of norethisterone:

1. **Breast Cancer**: Some studies have shown a slight increase in the risk of breast cancer with the use of hormonal contraceptives that contain synthetic progestins, including norethisterone. The risk appears to be related to the duration of use and tends to decrease after stopping the medication.

2. **Endometrial Cancer**: Hormonal contraceptives, including those containing norethisterone, have been found to reduce the risk of endometrial cancer. The protective effect is

attributed to the progestin component, which counteracts the proliferative effects of estrogen on the uterine lining.

3. **Ovarian Cancer**: Long-term use of hormonal contraceptives has been associated with a reduced risk of ovarian cancer. This protective effect is believed to result from the suppression of ovulation, reducing the number of times the ovarian epithelium is disrupted and repaired.

4. **Liver Cancer**: There is some evidence that long-term use of oral contraceptives may be associated with an increased risk of liver cancer, though this is less common and the data are less conclusive.

The overall risk of developing cancer from using norethisterone-containing products is generally considered low and must be weighed against the benefits of using these medications for contraception, menstrual regulation, and other therapeutic purposes. Healthcare providers assess individual risk factors when prescribing these medications to ensure the benefits outweigh the potential risks.

Trigger 86/101 – Oxymetholone

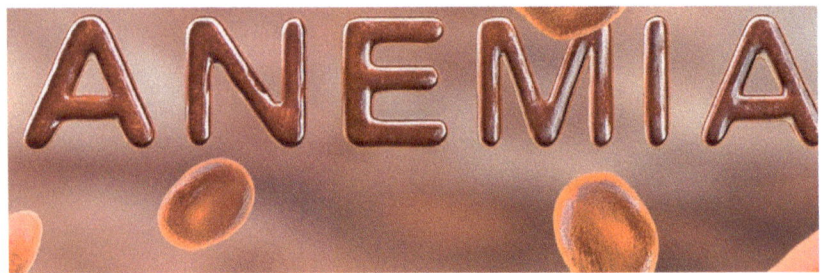

Report: 1st Report on Carcinogens
Category: chemical
Cancer Type(s): leukemia, liver cancer, esophageal

Oxymetholone, also known by its brand name Anadrol, is a synthetic anabolic steroid derived from dihydrotestosterone (DHT). It is primarily used in medicine to treat conditions such as anemia and osteoporosis, as well as to stimulate muscle growth in patients with muscle-wasting diseases. Additionally, oxymetholone is sometimes used illicitly by bodybuilders and athletes to enhance muscle mass and performance, although its use for such purposes is often associated with significant health risks.

Oxymetholone exerts its effects by binding to androgen receptors in the body, leading to increased protein synthesis, nitrogen retention, and red blood cell production. These actions contribute to its anabolic (muscle-building) and hematopoietic (blood-building) effects.

In medical settings, oxymetholone may be prescribed to stimulate muscle growth and weight gain in patients with conditions such as HIV/AIDS-associated wasting syndrome and severe burns. Oxymetholone is known to cause liver damage, including hepatotoxicity and cholestatic jaundice, particularly with long-term use or at high doses.

1. **Cardiovascular Effects**: Anabolic steroids like oxymetholone can increase the risk of cardiovascular complications, including hypertension, dyslipidemia, and thrombotic events.

2. **Endocrine Effects**: Oxymetholone can suppress the body's natural production of testosterone, leading to hormonal imbalances, testicular atrophy, and potential infertility.

3. **Virilization**: In women, oxymetholone use may cause virilizing effects such as deepening of the voice, enlargement of the clitoris, and development of male-pattern baldness.

Oxymetholone, like many other anabolic steroids, has been associated with an increased risk of certain types of cancer. However, it's essential to clarify that while there is evidence suggesting a potential link between anabolic steroid use and cancer, the exact mechanisms and extent of this association are not fully understood, and further research is needed.

Chronic use of anabolic steroids can disrupt the body's natural hormonal balance, including suppression of endogenous testosterone production and alterations in the levels of other hormones. Hormonal imbalances have been implicated in the development and progression of certain cancers, such as prostate cancer.

Some studies suggest that anabolic steroids may promote the growth of existing tumors by enhancing angiogenesis (formation of new blood vessels to support tumor growth) or suppressing immune responses against cancer cells.

Trigger 87/101 – Reserpine

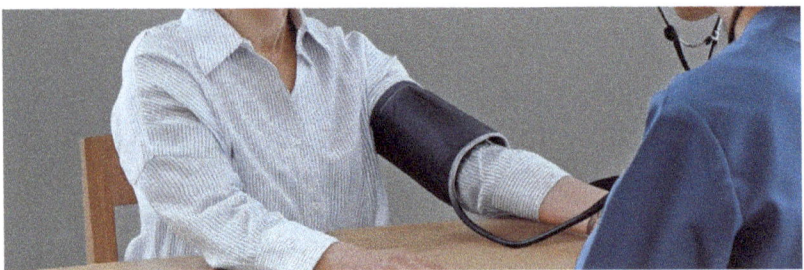

Report: 2nd Report on Carcinogens
Category: chemical
Cancer Type(s): breast

Reserpine is a naturally occurring indole alkaloid derived from the roots of certain plant species, including Rauwolfia serpentina and Rauwolfia vomitoria. It is best known for its antipsychotic and antihypertensive properties and has been used in medicine for the treatment of various conditions, including hypertension, psychosis, and certain behavioral disorders.

Medical uses include:

1. **Hypertension**: Reserpine was historically used as an antihypertensive medication to treat high blood pressure (hypertension). It was particularly useful in the management of essential hypertension.

2. **Psychosis**: Reserpine was also used as an antipsychotic medication to treat various psychotic disorders, including schizophrenia. It was one of the first medications introduced for the treatment of psychosis.

Reserpine can affect hormone levels, leading to symptoms such as breast enlargement (gynecomastia) and impotence.

Unraveling the Origins: Exploring 101 Triggers of Cancer

Reserpine is a naturally occurring indole alkaloid with antipsychotic and antihypertensive properties. While it was historically used in the treatment of hypertension and psychosis, its use has declined in modern medicine due to its side effects and the availability of alternative medications. However, it remains an important compound in the history of pharmacology and the development of antipsychotic and antihypertensive drugs.

Trigger 88/101 – Selenium Sulfide

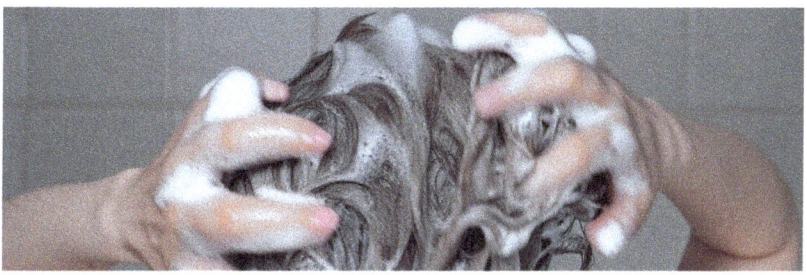

Report: 3rd Report on Carcinogens
Category: chemical
Cancer Type(s): liver, lung

Selenium sulfide is primarily used in the treatment of dandruff and certain fungal infections of the skin, scalp, and other areas of the body. Selenium sulfide is known for its antifungal and antimitotic properties, which help to control the growth of fungi and reduce inflammation associated with conditions such as dandruff and seborrheic dermatitis.

Key Properties and Information:

1. **Chemical Structure**: Selenium sulfide is composed of selenium and sulfur atoms arranged in a crystalline structure. It is

available in various formulations, including suspensions, shampoos, lotions, and creams, for topical application.

2. **Antifungal Action**: Selenium sulfide exerts its antifungal effects by inhibiting the growth and reproduction of fungi, including Malassezia species, which are implicated in the development of dandruff and seborrheic dermatitis. It disrupts the fungal cell membrane, interferes with fungal metabolism, and inhibits fungal replication.

Selenium sulfide may also be used in the treatment of other fungal skin infections, such as tinea versicolor (pityriasis versicolor), a superficial fungal infection characterized by discolored patches on the skin.

Selenium sulfide's antifungal activity is attributed to its ability to inhibit enzymes involved in fungal metabolism, disrupt membrane function, and interfere with nucleic acid synthesis. These actions lead to the suppression of fungal growth and the alleviation of associated symptoms.

While there are other antifungal agents available for similar purposes, selenium sulfide continues to be a preferred choice for many individuals and healthcare professionals due to its efficacy and established track record in managing dandruff and related conditions. It is available over-the-counter in various formulations, including shampoos, lotions, and creams, making it accessible to consumers seeking relief from dandruff and fungal skin infections.

Unraveling the Origins: Exploring 101 Triggers of Cancer

Trigger 89/101 – Vinyl Bromide

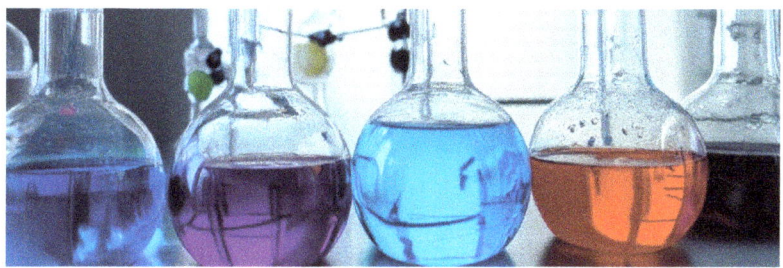

Report: 10th Report on Carcinogens
Category: chemical
Cancer Type(s): liver

Vinyl bromide, also known as bromoethene, is primarily used as an intermediate in the production of various organic compounds. It can be used to synthesize brominated polymers, which have applications in fire retardants and other specialty materials. It is also used in the synthesis of copolymers and as a building block in the manufacture of pharmaceuticals and agrochemicals.

Vinyl bromide is toxic and poses health risks if inhaled. Acute exposure can cause respiratory irritation, dizziness, headache, and other symptoms. Chronic exposure may have more serious health effects. Vinyl bromide is classified as a possible human carcinogen (Group 2A) by the International Agency for Research on Cancer (IARC) based on evidence from animal studies. Long-term exposure to vinyl bromide has been associated with an increased risk of developing liver cancer and other tumors in laboratory animals.

Vinyl bromide is a valuable chemical intermediate used in the synthesis of various organic compounds, particularly in polymer and pharmaceutical production.

Vinyl bromide, primarily used as an intermediate in organic synthesis, can be involved in the production of various pharmaceuticals and agrochemicals. However, it is not typically a final active ingredient in these products but rather a building block used in the chemical synthesis of more complex compounds. Here are some examples of its applications:

Pharmaceuticals:

1. **Synthesis of Active Pharmaceutical Ingredients (APIs):** Vinyl bromide is used in the synthesis of APIs through various organic reactions, including polymerization and substitution reactions. It helps introduce vinyl groups into more complex molecules.

2. **Intermediate in Drug Synthesis:** It can be a starting material or an intermediate in the synthesis of several classes of pharmaceuticals, including:

   - **Antiviral agents:** Certain antiviral drugs require vinyl or bromine-containing intermediates during their synthesis.
   - **Anticancer agents:** Some chemotherapeutic agents are synthesized using vinyl bromide as an intermediate to introduce specific functional groups into the drug molecules.
   - **Anti-inflammatory drugs:** Used in the synthesis of specific NSAIDs (Non-Steroidal Anti-Inflammatory Drugs).

Agrochemicals:

1. **Pesticides and Herbicides:** Vinyl bromide is used in the synthesis of various pesticides and herbicides. It helps create molecules that can disrupt the biological processes of pests and weeds.

- **Insecticides**: Some insecticides are synthesized using vinyl bromide as a precursor to introduce functional groups that are effective against insect pests.
- **Fungicides**: Certain fungicides, which protect crops from fungal infections, may also involve vinyl bromide in their synthesis.

2. **Plant Growth Regulators**: Vinyl bromide can be used to synthesize compounds that act as plant growth regulators, influencing the growth and development of crops.

Vinyl bromide is an important chemical intermediate used in the synthesis of a wide range of pharmaceuticals and agrochemicals. Its role is critical in introducing specific functional groups into complex molecules, which are then further processed to produce active compounds used in medicine and agriculture. Due to its reactivity and usefulness in organic synthesis, it remains a valuable tool in the chemical industry despite the need for careful handling and safety measures due to its toxic and potentially carcinogenic properties.

Trigger 90/101 – Tris(2,3-dibromopropyl) Phosphate

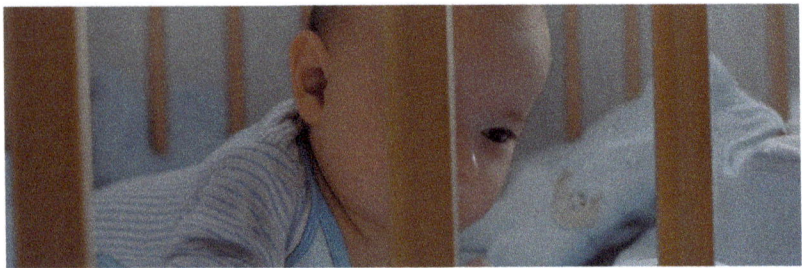

Report: 2nd Report on Carcinogens
Category: chemical
Cancer Type(s): liver

Tris(2,3-dibromopropyl) phosphate (TDBPP), also known as tris(2,3-dibromopropyl)phosphate or simply "tris," was widely used as a flame retardant in various consumer products, particularly in children's sleepwear, textiles, polyurethane foams, and plastics. Its purpose was to reduce the flammability of these materials and enhance fire safety.

TDBPP has been found to be toxic, with potential effects on the liver and kidneys. It can also cause skin and eye irritation upon contact. Research, particularly animal studies, has indicated that TDBPP is a carcinogen. It has been shown to cause cancer in laboratory animals, leading to significant health concerns regarding its use. TDBPP has also been shown to be mutagenic, meaning it can cause changes to the genetic material in cells, which can lead to cancer.

Due to its carcinogenic and mutagenic properties, TDBPP has been banned or restricted in many countries. For example, it was banned from use in children's sleepwear in the United States in the late 1970s following studies that demonstrated its potential to cause cancer. However, TDBPP is persistent in the environment and can accumulate in living organisms, raising concerns about its long-term ecological impact.

In addition to children's sleepwear, it has been using in the following:

1. **Upholstered Furniture**: TDBPP has been used in upholstered furniture, including sofas, chairs, and mattresses, to meet flammability standards and regulations. Polyurethane foam, a common component of upholstered furniture, is often treated with flame retardants to reduce the risk of fire-related accidents.

2. **Textiles and Fabrics**: TDBPP was used in textiles and fabrics to impart flame retardant properties. This application is particularly relevant in products such as curtains, carpets, upholstery fabrics, and draperies, where fire safety considerations are important.

3. **Electronics**: Flame retardants, including TDBPP, have been used in electronic devices and appliances to mitigate fire hazards associated with electrical malfunctions or overheating. They may be incorporated into plastic casings, circuit boards, and other components to reduce the risk of fire and enhance product safety.

4. **Automotive Interiors**: TDBPP might have been used in automotive interiors, such as car seats, dashboard components, and upholstery materials, to improve fire resistance and comply with automotive safety standards.

5. **Building Materials**: Flame retardants, including TDBPP, have been used in construction materials, such as insulation foams, wall coverings, and roofing materials, to enhance fire safety in residential and commercial buildings.

In response to health concerns and regulatory actions, the use of TDBPP and other brominated flame retardants has decreased significantly in many consumer products. Bans, restrictions, and voluntary phase-outs have been implemented in various countries to limit exposure to these chemicals and promote the use of safer alternatives.

As a result, manufacturers have increasingly shifted towards alternative flame retardants and fire safety strategies that prioritize efficacy, sustainability, and human health considerations. This transition reflects ongoing efforts to balance fire safety requirements with environmental and health concerns associated with chemical additives like TDBPP.

Trigger 91/101 – Toxaphene

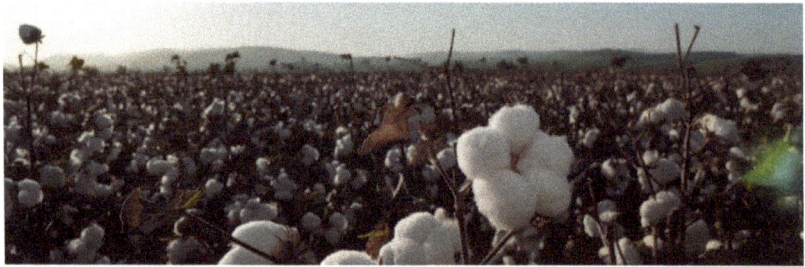

Report: 2nd Report on Carcinogens
Category: chemical
Cancer Type(s): nonHodgkin lymphoma , leukemia

Toxaphene is a complex mixture of polychlorinated camphene derivatives that was once widely used as an insecticide. It was primarily used to control pests in agriculture, including insects such as cotton bollworms, caterpillars, and various pests in crops like cotton, fruits, vegetables, and grains. Toxaphene was also used in public health programs to combat pests such as mosquitoes. It disrupts the function of neurotransmitters in insects, leading to paralysis and death.

Toxaphene is highly persistent in the environment, resisting degradation by sunlight, water, and microorganisms. It can persist in soil, water, and sediments for long periods, leading to potential bioaccumulation in food chains. Its persistence and ability to travel long distances through air and water currents have led to its widespread distribution in ecosystems, even in regions where it was not directly applied.

Toxaphene is highly toxic to humans and animals. Exposure to toxaphene can cause acute poisoning symptoms such as nausea, vomiting, dizziness, and seizures. Long-term exposure may lead to chronic health effects, including neurological, reproductive, and developmental disorders. Toxaphene is classified as a probable human carcinogen by the International Agency for Research on Cancer (IARC), based on animal studies showing an increased incidence of cancer, particularly liver tumors, in exposed animals.

Toxaphene has been banned or severely restricted in many countries due to its significant health and environmental risks. The Stockholm Convention on Persistent Organic Pollutants (POPs) lists toxaphene as a POP, aiming to eliminate or reduce its production, use, and release into the environment.

The Environmental Protection Agency (EPA) took regulatory action to cancel the registration of toxaphene for all uses in the United States in 1990 due to concerns about its persistence, toxicity, and environmental impact. This action effectively prohibited the manufacture, distribution, sale, and use of toxaphene-containing products in the country

Trigger 92/101 – Cyclophosphamide

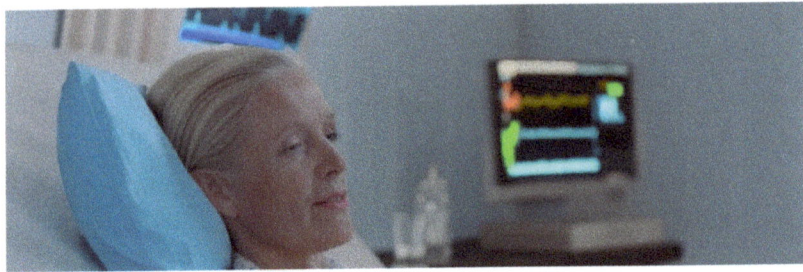

Report: 2nd Report on Carcinogens
Category: chemical
Cancer Type(s): nonHodgkin lymphoma , leukemia

Cyclophosphamide is a chemotherapy medication used to treat various types of cancer and autoimmune diseases. It belongs to a class of drugs known as alkylating agents, which work by interfering with the DNA replication process in rapidly dividing cells, ultimately leading to cell death.

Cyclophosphamide is a prodrug, meaning it undergoes chemical changes in the body to form its active metabolites, including phosphoramide mustard and acrolein. Phosphoramide mustard is the primary active metabolite responsible for the cytotoxic effects of cyclophosphamide. It crosslinks DNA strands, inhibiting DNA synthesis and leading to cell death. Acrolein is a toxic metabolite that can cause bladder irritation and hemorrhagic cystitis. Mesna, a drug that helps protect the bladder lining, is often administered with cyclophosphamide to reduce the risk of bladder toxicity.

Cyclophosphamide is used to treat various types of cancer, including leukemia, lymphoma, multiple myeloma, breast cancer, ovarian cancer, and certain types of solid tumors. It is also used in the treatment of autoimmune diseases, such as rheumatoid arthritis, systemic lupus erythematosus (SLE), and vasculitis. In these conditions, cyclophosphamide works by suppressing the overactive immune system.

Cyclophosphamide is still used today in the treatment of various types of cancer and autoimmune diseases. Despite the development of newer chemotherapy drugs and targeted therapies, cyclophosphamide remains an important component of treatment regimens. Cyclophosphamide is a relatively inexpensive chemotherapy agent compared to some newer targeted therapies, making it an attractive option in settings where cost is a consideration.

While newer treatments continue to emerge, cyclophosphamide remains an essential component of cancer and autoimmune disease treatment regimens, particularly in situations where it is known to be effective or where alternatives may not be readily available or affordable.

Trigger 93/101 – Azathioprine

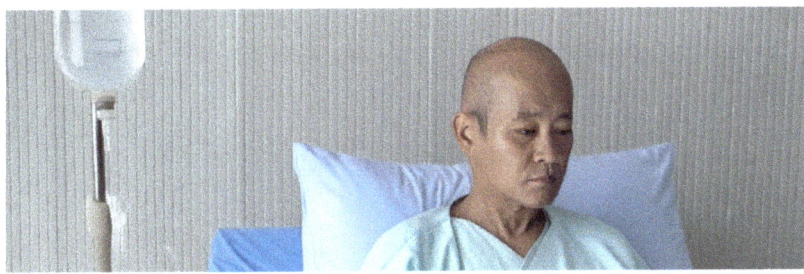

Report: 4th Report on Carcinogens
Category: chemical
Cancer Type(s): nonHodgkin lymphoma, skin, liver

Azathioprine is an immunosuppressive medication used primarily to prevent organ rejection after transplantation and to treat certain autoimmune diseases. It is classified as a purine analog, meaning it interferes with the synthesis of DNA and RNA, ultimately suppressing the immune system's response.

Azathioprine is metabolized in the body to form 6-mercaptopurine (6-MP), which is further converted into active metabolites that interfere with the synthesis of DNA and RNA. By inhibiting the proliferation of rapidly dividing immune cells, azathioprine suppresses the immune response, making it useful in preventing rejection of transplanted organs and in treating autoimmune diseases where the immune system attacks the body's tissues.

Azathioprine is still currently being used today in the treatment of various medical conditions. Azathioprine is a relatively inexpensive medication compared to some newer immunosuppressive agents, making it an attractive option in healthcare settings where cost is a consideration.

Trigger 94/101 – Malathion

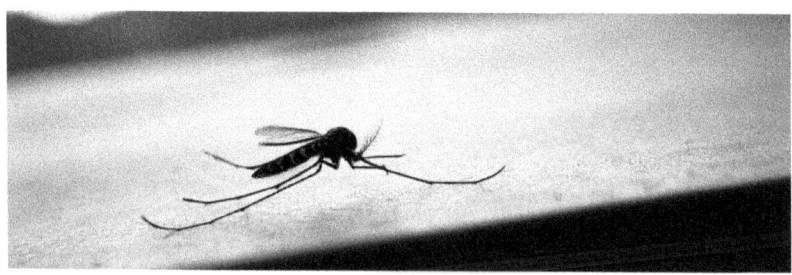

Report: NCI Technical Report Series No. 24
Category: chemical
Cancer Type(s): mammary

Unraveling the Origins: Exploring 101 Triggers of Cancer

Malathion is an organophosphate insecticide commonly used in agriculture, public health programs, and residential pest control to control a wide range of insects, including mosquitoes, flies, ants, and agricultural pests. While malathion has been classified by some regulatory agencies as having the potential to cause cancer, the evidence regarding its carcinogenicity is mixed and subject to ongoing debate.

The International Agency for Research on Cancer (IARC), a specialized agency of the World Health Organization (WHO), has classified malathion as "probably carcinogenic to humans" (Group 2A) based on limited evidence in humans and sufficient evidence in animals. This classification was based on studies indicating an increased incidence of certain cancers, particularly leukemia, in laboratory animals exposed to high doses of malathion.

Overall, the carcinogenicity of malathion remains a topic of scientific debate, and regulatory agencies continue to monitor new research and conduct risk assessments to inform regulatory decisions. While some studies have suggested a potential link between malathion exposure and cancer risk, the evidence is not conclusive, and further research is needed to better understand the potential health effects of malathion and other organophosphate pesticides.

Malathion is sometimes used to treat head lice infestations, although it is not the first-line treatment option in many regions. Malathion lotion is available by prescription in some countries for the treatment of head lice, particularly when other treatments have failed or when resistance to other treatments is suspected.

Malathion lotion works by disrupting the nervous system of lice and their eggs (nits), leading to their death. It is typically applied to dry hair and left on for a specified period before being washed out. Repeat treatments may be necessary to ensure that all lice and nits are eradicated.

Trigger 95/101 – Glyphosate

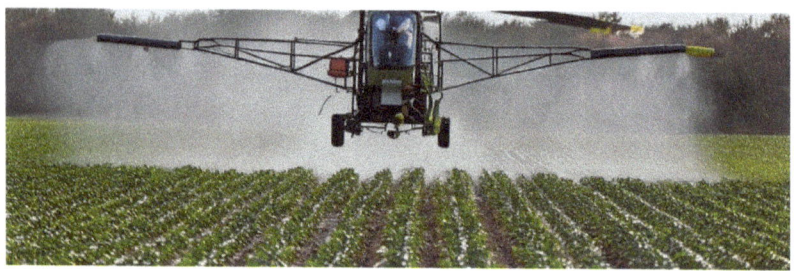

Report: IARC 2015
Category: chemical
Cancer Type(s): skin, liver

Glyphosate is a broad-spectrum herbicide widely used to kill weeds, especially annual broadleaf weeds and grasses that compete with crops. It was first introduced in the 1970s and has become one of the most widely used herbicides globally. Glyphosate works by inhibiting an enzyme pathway essential for plant growth, effectively causing plants to wither and die. It is commonly applied in agriculture, forestry, urban landscaping, and home gardening to control weeds and improve crop yields. Glyphosate is also used as a desiccant to accelerate the drying process of certain crops before harvest. However, its use has been controversial due to concerns about its potential impact on human health, wildlife, and the environment.

The classification of glyphosate as a carcinogen has been a topic of significant debate and controversy among scientists, regulatory agencies, and advocacy groups worldwide.

Unraveling the Origins: Exploring 101 Triggers of Cancer

In 2015, the IARC, a specialized agency of the World Health Organization (WHO), classified glyphosate as "probably carcinogenic to humans" (Group 2A) based on limited evidence in humans and sufficient evidence in experimental animals. The classification was primarily based on studies suggesting an association between glyphosate exposure and an increased risk of non-Hodgkin lymphoma (NHL) in humans and animals.

The EPA, responsible for regulating pesticides in the United States, has conducted multiple assessments of glyphosate's carcinogenic potential. In 2017, the EPA released a draft risk assessment concluding that glyphosate is not likely to be carcinogenic to humans. However, this assessment was met with criticism from some scientists and advocacy groups who argued that the EPA's conclusions did not adequately consider all available evidence.

The European Food Safety Authority (EFSA), responsible for evaluating the safety of pesticides in the European Union, has also conducted assessments of glyphosate's carcinogenic potential. In 2015, the EFSA concluded that glyphosate is unlikely to pose a carcinogenic hazard to humans. However, this conclusion was challenged by the IARC's classification and led to further debate within the scientific community.

Overall, while there is ongoing debate and controversy surrounding glyphosate's carcinogenicity, regulatory agencies and scientific bodies continue to evaluate the available evidence and conduct risk assessments to inform regulatory decisions. The classification of glyphosate as a carcinogen varies depending on the criteria and evidence considered by different organizations, highlighting the complexity of assessing the health risks associated with pesticide exposure.

Trigger 96/101 – Glycidol

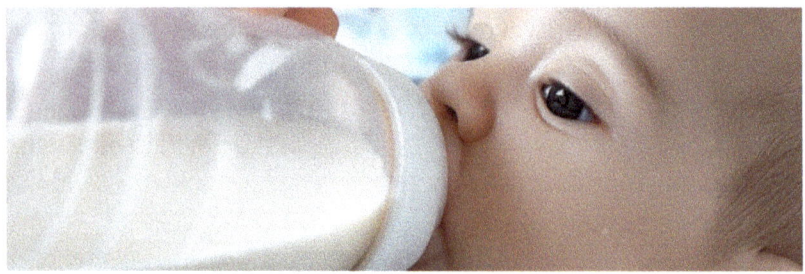

Report: 7th Report on Carcinogens
Category: chemical
Cancer Type(s): mammary, brain, uterus, liver

Glycidol has been classified as a probable human carcinogen by the International Agency for Research on Cancer (IARC) based on animal studies showing that exposure to glycidol can cause tumors, particularly in the liver and lung. Additionally, glycidol has been shown to have mutagenic and genotoxic effects, meaning it can damage DNA and increase the risk of cancer.

Due to its carcinogenic properties, glycidol exposure in occupational settings is regulated, and measures are taken to minimize worker exposure to this chemical. In consumer products, glycidol and its derivatives are subject to regulations and may have restrictions on their use in certain applications to protect public health and safety.

Lycidyl esters, which can degrade into glycidol, have been detected in certain infant formula products. Glycidyl esters can form in edible oils during refining processes, particularly when oils are exposed to high temperatures and pressures.

When glycidyl esters are present in food products, such as refined vegetable oils, they can potentially degrade into glycidol during food processing or storage, especially under conditions of heat or acidic pH.

Concerns about the presence of glycidyl esters and glycidol in food products, including infant formula, have prompted regulatory agencies and food manufacturers to take measures to minimize exposure. Some regulatory agencies have set limits or guidelines for glycidyl esters in food products, and manufacturers may use alternative refining processes or select oils with lower levels of glycidyl esters to reduce the risk of glycidol formation.

It's important to note that the presence of glycidol or its precursors in infant formula is a concern because infants are particularly vulnerable to the potential health effects of carcinogenic compounds. Therefore, regulatory agencies and food manufacturers are vigilant in monitoring and minimizing the presence of glycidyl esters and glycidol in infant formula and other food products consumed by infants and young children.

Trigger 97/101 – Ciclosporin

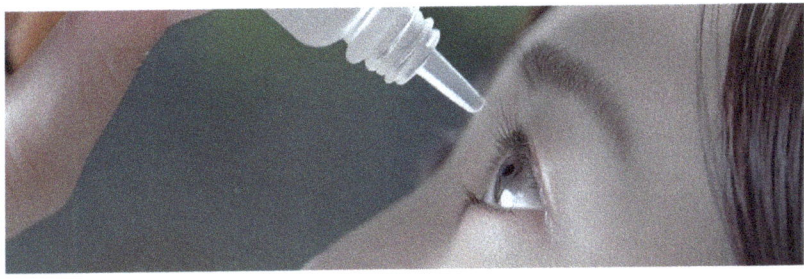

Report: 8th Report on Carcinogens
Category: chemical
Cancer Type(s): lymphoma, Kaposi, sarcoma, or skin cancer

Ciclosporin, also known as cyclosporine, is an immunosuppressant medication commonly used to prevent organ rejection in transplant patients. It is also used to treat various autoimmune conditions, such as rheumatoid arthritis, psoriasis, and certain chronic eye conditions. Ciclosporin works by inhibiting the activity of T-lymphocytes, which are a type of white blood cell involved in the immune response.

Ciclosporin is classified as a carcinogen primarily because of its immunosuppressive properties, which can increase the risk of developing cancer. Here are the main reasons why Ciclosporin is considered a carcinogen:

1. **Immunosuppression**: Ciclosporin suppresses the immune system to prevent organ rejection and to treat autoimmune diseases. A suppressed immune system is less capable of detecting and destroying cancer cells, which can lead to an increased risk of cancer development.

2. **Increased Risk of Lymphomas and Skin Cancers**: Long-term use of Ciclosporin has been associated with a higher incidence of lymphomas (a type of blood cancer) and skin cancers. This is particularly evident in transplant patients who require chronic immunosuppression to prevent organ rejection.

3. **Genotoxic Effects**: Some studies suggest that Ciclosporin may have genotoxic effects, meaning it can cause damage to the genetic material within cells, leading to mutations and potentially to cancer development.

4. **Proliferation of Oncogenic Viruses**: Ciclosporin use can promote the proliferation of oncogenic viruses (viruses that can cause cancer), such as the Epstein-Barr virus, which is linked to certain types of lymphoma.

5. **Tumor Growth Promotion**: There is evidence that Ciclosporin may directly promote the growth of existing cancer cells by influencing various cellular pathways involved in cell proliferation and survival.

Due to these factors, patients taking Ciclosporin are closely monitored for signs of cancer, and the benefits and risks of the medication are carefully weighed by healthcare providers. It's important for patients on Ciclosporin to follow their healthcare provider's recommendations and to undergo regular screenings for early detection of any potential malignancies.

Trigger 98/101 – N-Nitrosodimethylamine

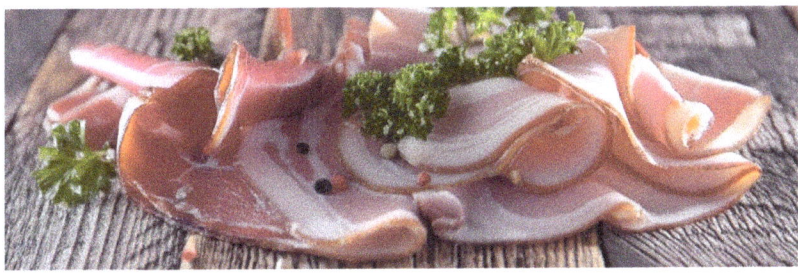

Report: 6th Report on Carcinogens
Category: chemical
Cancer Type(s): stomach, small/large intestine

N-Nitrosodimethylamine (NDMA) is known to be a contaminant in various food products, drinking water, and certain pharmaceuticals. NDMA is classified as a probable human carcinogen by the International Agency for Research on Cancer (IARC). It has been shown to cause cancer in various animal studies and is believed to pose a similar risk to humans.

NDMA can form during the manufacturing process of certain pharmaceuticals, from the degradation of dimethylhydrazine (a rocket fuel), and as a byproduct of chlorination in water treatment. It can also be found in smoked or cured meats, beer, and tobacco smoke. Exposure to NDMA can increase the risk of developing various types of cancer, including liver, kidney, and gastrointestinal cancers. Acute exposure can cause liver damage, nausea, vomiting, and other symptoms of toxicity.

NDMA has been in the news due to contamination issues in certain medications, such as ranitidine (Zantac) and some blood pressure drugs (sartans). These contaminants have led to recalls and increased scrutiny of manufacturing processes to prevent NDMA formation.

Understanding and mitigating exposure to NDMA is important for public health, given its potent carcinogenic properties.

Trigger 99/101 – Benzene

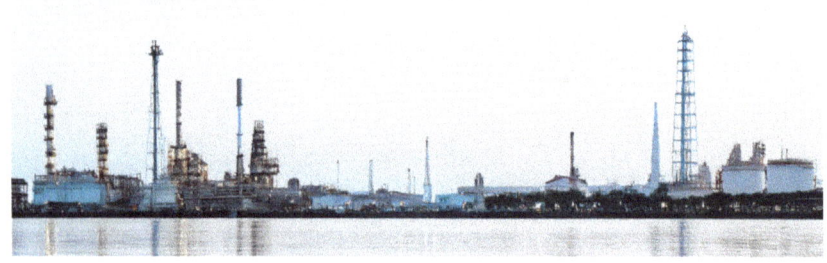

Report: 1st Report on Carcinogens
Carcinogen Category: environment
Cancer Type(s): leukemia, lung, skin

Unraveling the Origins: Exploring 101 Triggers of Cancer

Benzene is a colorless, flammable liquid with a sweet odor. It is a natural component of crude oil and is also produced as a byproduct in various industrial processes, including petroleum refining and the production of certain chemicals. Benzene is one of the most widely used chemicals in the United States, with applications in the manufacturing of plastics, synthetic fibers, rubber, dyes, detergents, pesticides, and many other products.

While benzene has many industrial uses, it is also a known carcinogen. Long-term exposure to benzene can cause serious health effects, including leukemia and other cancers of the blood-forming organs, such as bone marrow and lymphatic system. Benzene can enter the body through inhalation, ingestion, or absorption through the skin. It is metabolized in the liver and can affect the production of blood cells and damage DNA.

Due to its carcinogenic properties, benzene exposure in the workplace is regulated by occupational safety agencies, and permissible exposure limits have been established to protect workers. In addition to occupational exposure, benzene can also be found in low levels in ambient air due to emissions from industrial sources, vehicle exhaust, and cigarette smoke.

Benzene can be found in various products and substances due to its widespread use in industrial processes and manufacturing. Some common products and sources of benzene include:

1. **Petroleum Products**: Benzene is a natural component of crude oil and is present in various petroleum-derived products, including gasoline, diesel fuel, automobile exhaust, industrial emissions, and fuel evaporation from gasoline filling stations.

2. **Plastics**: Benzene is used in the production of plastics, including polystyrene, styrene-butadiene rubber (SBR), and polyethylene. It is a key ingredient in the production of

styrene, which is used to make polystyrene plastics and synthetic rubber.

3. **Synthetic Fibers**: Benzene is used in the manufacture of synthetic fibers such as nylon and polyester.

4. **Rubber**: Benzene is used in the production of rubber, including synthetic rubber and rubber additives.

5. **Dyes and Pigments**: Benzene is used as a solvent in the production of dyes, pigments, and other colorants used in paints, inks, and coatings.

6. **Adhesives and Sealants**: Benzene is used as a solvent in the production of adhesives, sealants, and coatings.

7. **Pesticides and Herbicides**: Benzene is used as an intermediate in the production of certain pesticides and herbicides.

8. **Cleaning Products**: Benzene may be found in certain cleaning products and solvents used for degreasing and other industrial applications.

9. **Cigarette Smoke**: Benzene is present in cigarette smoke as a byproduct of tobacco combustion.

10. **Automotive Products**: Benzene may be present in automotive products such as motor oil, brake fluid, and antifreeze.

11. **Consumer Products**: Benzene has also been found in some consumer products, including hand sanitizers and sun-care products.

Unraveling the Origins: Exploring 101 Triggers of Cancer

Consumers can reduce their exposure to benzene by following safety guidelines and choosing products that are manufactured with benzene-free alternatives when possible.

Trigger 100/101 – Butylated hydroxyanisole (BHA)

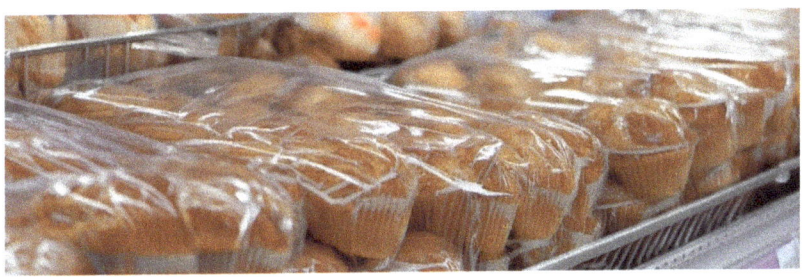

Report: 6th Report on Carcinogens
Category: chemical
Cancer Type(s): stomach

Butylated hydroxyanisole (BHA) is a synthetic antioxidant commonly used as a food preservative to prevent the oxidation of fats and oils, which helps extend shelf life and maintain product quality.

BHA is widely used as a preservative in various foods, including baked goods, snacks, meats, cereals, chewing gum, and fats/oils. Its primary function is to prevent rancidity and maintain flavor and color stability.

It is also used in cosmetics, pharmaceuticals, rubber, and petroleum products to prevent oxidation and extend shelf life. BHA is used in animal feed to protect the nutritional quality of the feed.

BHA works by scavenging free radicals and decomposing peroxides, which are products of lipid oxidation. By interrupting the oxidation process, BHA helps preserve the integrity and quality of food and other products.

Despite its approved status, there has been some controversy over the potential health effects of BHA. Animal studies have shown that high doses can cause certain health issues, such as liver and thyroid effects, and there is some evidence suggesting it may be a carcinogen in animals.

Long-term studies in animals, primarily rats and mice, have shown that high doses of BHA can lead to the development of tumors. Specifically, these studies have found an increased incidence of forestomach tumors in rodents fed high levels of BHA. These findings are significant because they indicate that BHA has the potential to induce carcinogenic effects in laboratory animals when consumed in large amounts over extended periods.

BHA can induce oxidative stress and generate reactive oxygen species (ROS) during its metabolic processing in the body. These ROS can cause damage to cellular components, including DNA, proteins, and lipids, leading to mutations and other cellular changes associated with cancer development.

In summary, BHA is considered a potential carcinogen primarily based on animal studies showing that high doses can lead to tumor development. The mechanisms involving oxidative stress and genetic alterations further support its classification as a possible carcinogen.

Unraveling the Origins: Exploring 101 Triggers of Cancer

Trigger 101/101 – Isobutyl Nitrite

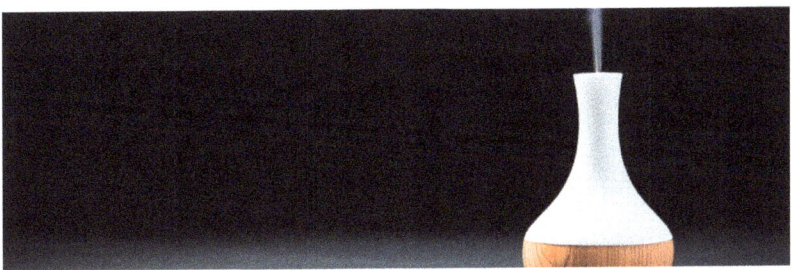

Report: NIH Publication No. 96-3364
Category: chemical
Cancer Type(s): esophageal, gastric, and liver

Isobutyl nitrite belongs to a class of chemicals known as alkyl nitrites, which are also referred to as "poppers" in common parlance. Isobutyl nitrite is primarily known for its use as a recreational drug and in some industrial applications.

Here are some key points about isobutyl nitrite:

1. **Recreational Use**: Isobutyl nitrite, like other alkyl nitrites, is often used recreationally to produce a brief but intense rush or high. It is inhaled, typically by inhaling vapors from an opened bottle, leading to muscle relaxation and a feeling of euphoria.

2. **Vasodilator**: Isobutyl nitrite is a potent vasodilator, meaning it dilates blood vessels. This property can cause a drop in blood pressure and increase blood flow to various parts of the body, including the brain.

3. **Legal Status**: The legal status of isobutyl nitrite varies by jurisdiction. In some places, it is regulated as a controlled substance due to its recreational use and health risks.

4. **Health Risks**: Misuse or excessive inhalation can lead to adverse effects such as dizziness, headaches, nausea, and in severe cases, methemoglobinemia (a condition where oxygen is unable to bind to hemoglobin effectively). Prolonged or frequent use can also lead to tolerance and dependency.

5. **Industrial Use**: Isobutyl nitrite has industrial applications as a solvent, a precursor in chemical synthesis, and as a reagent in certain chemical reactions.

Isobutyl nitrite is primarily known for its use in recreational products rather than commercial consumer goods. It is commonly found in products labeled as "room odorants," "leather cleaners," "video head cleaners," and similar euphemistic names. These products are marketed in a way that avoids directly referencing their recreational use due to legal restrictions.

It is important to note that the use of isobutyl nitrite in these products is primarily intended for its recreational effects, even though they are labeled for other purposes to circumvent legal restrictions.

The sale and distribution of isobutyl nitrite-containing products are subject to regulatory scrutiny in many jurisdictions due to health risks associated with their misuse. As such, they are often found in specialty shops, adult stores, and online marketplaces that cater to recreational users.

Unraveling the Origins: Exploring 101 Triggers of Cancer

CHAPTER 14: EXAMINING THE TRIGGERS

The chart below illustrates that the Chemical category dominates the triggers that cause cancer. Consequently, most causes of cancer are indeed linked to human activities. Only a few cancer risk factors are beyond human control; however, many can be mitigated through lifestyle changes and preventive measures.

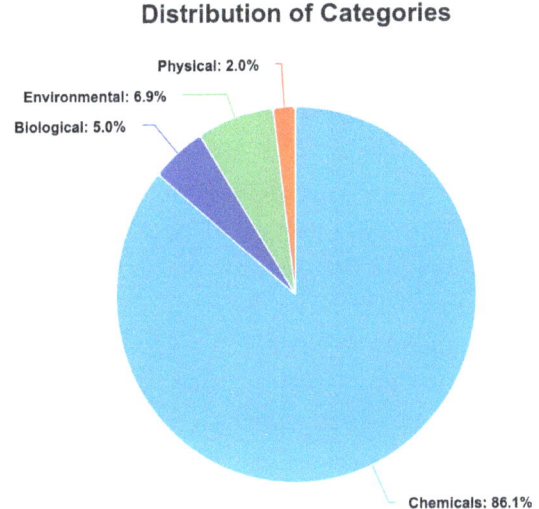

The breakdown of the triggers listed are as follows:

- **Chemical**: 87
- **Biology**: 5
- **Environment**: 7
- **Physical**: 2

Most of the triggers are oil byproducts which are linked to cancer primarily due to the presence of hazardous chemicals and pollutants associated with their extraction, refinement, and use. Carcinogenic substances such as benzene, toluene, xylene, and polycyclic aromatic hydrocarbons (PAHs) are often found in these byproducts, significantly increasing cancer risk. The burning of fossil fuels, a major source of oil byproducts, releases pollutants like particulate matter and volatile organic compounds into the air, which can contribute to respiratory issues and a higher risk of lung cancer over time. Workers in the oil and gas industry face increased cancer risk due to exposure to harmful chemicals and pollutants, including substances like asbestos in older facilities and various chemicals used in drilling and refining processes. Additionally, environmental contamination from oil spills and leaks can lead to soil and water pollution, raising cancer risk for communities in affected areas. Chemical residues from oil-derived products, such as certain pesticides and industrial chemicals, can also contribute to cancer risk through prolonged exposure. Addressing these risks involves regulatory measures to control emissions, improve industry safety practices, and minimize personal exposure to contaminated environments.

Many plastics are made from byproducts of oil. Plastics pose significant hazards to human health primarily due to their chemical composition and environmental interactions. Many plastics contain harmful additives, such as plasticizers, flame retardants, and stabilizers, which can be toxic. As plastics degrade, they form microplastics—tiny particles that can be ingested or inhaled, potentially leading to inflammation or other health problems. Additionally, plastics can leach harmful chemicals into food, beverages, or the environment, especially when exposed to heat or acidic conditions. The environmental contamination caused by plastics can also have indirect health effects, such as respiratory issues and cardiovascular diseases, due to polluted air, water, and soil. The persistent nature of plastics in the environment further exacerbates these risks, as accumulated plastic waste can lead to prolonged exposure to hazardous chemicals. Reducing plastic use, improving waste management, and opting for safer materials can help mitigate these health risks.

Before plastics became widespread, products were primarily made from natural materials and metals. Wood was commonly used for furniture, tools, utensils, and construction due to its versatility and availability. Metals like iron, steel, and aluminum were employed in tools, kitchenware, machinery, and building structures, valued for their durability and strength. Glass was a popular material for containers, windows, and decorative items because of its durability and ability to be molded into various shapes. Ceramics and pottery were utilized for dishes, cookware, tiles, and art, prized for their heat resistance and versatility. Leather was used for clothing, shoes, belts, and accessories, appreciated for its durability and flexibility. Textiles made from natural fibers such as cotton, wool, silk, and linen were employed in clothing, upholstery, and other fabric products. Natural rubber, derived from rubber tree sap, was used in tires, boots, and various industrial goods before synthetic rubber became common. Additionally, materials like bone, horn, and shell were used in tools, jewelry, and decorative items. These materials were chosen for their properties and suitability, reflecting the technological and material constraints of their times.

CHAPTER 15: FINAL THOUGHTS

I firmly believe that the incidence of cancer can be significantly reduced by understanding and eliminating the triggers that contribute to its development from our daily lives. We must take personal responsibility for our health and not rely on others to address what we are unwilling to address ourselves.

"Knowing is half the battle" is a phrase that emphasizes the importance of awareness and knowledge as crucial components of success and problem-solving. This adage suggests that being informed about a situation, potential challenges, or the tools available to address them is a significant step toward achieving a desired outcome. When people have a clear understanding of what they are facing, they can make more informed decisions, anticipate obstacles, and strategize effectively. This concept is often applied in various contexts, from education and professional development to personal growth and crisis management.

The phrase gained popular recognition from the 1980s animated TV series "G.I. Joe," where it was used as a tagline at the end of educational segments, "Now you know, and knowing is half the battle." In a broader sense, it underscores the value of learning and preparation. By acquiring knowledge, individuals can demystify complex issues, reduce uncertainty, and build confidence. This proactive approach helps to mitigate risks and enhances the ability to navigate challenges efficiently. Ultimately, while knowledge alone may not solve all problems, it provides a foundation that empowers individuals to take meaningful action and improve their chances of success.

While "knowing is half the battle," the other half involves taking action based on that knowledge. This concept highlights that awareness and understanding are essential, but they must be followed by practical steps to achieve goals and resolve issues.

Unraveling the Origins: Exploring 101 Triggers of Cancer

The transition from knowledge to action encompasses planning, decision-making, and execution. It requires discipline, persistence, and often creativity to apply what one knows effectively in real-world situations.

Taking action is where many challenges arise, as it involves navigating uncertainties, adapting to changing circumstances, and overcoming obstacles. This phase requires not only physical or mental effort but also emotional resilience and a willingness to engage with difficulties. For example, in a workplace setting, knowing the best practices for a project is crucial, but it's the implementation of these practices—managing teams, meeting deadlines, and adapting to feedback—that ultimately determines success. Similarly, in personal development, understanding the principles of a healthy lifestyle is important, but it is the consistent application of healthy habits that leads to meaningful change.

The interplay between knowledge and action is dynamic and ongoing. It involves continuous learning, as taking action often provides new insights and experiences that inform future decisions. This cyclical process of gaining knowledge and acting upon it is fundamental to growth and progress in any field. Therefore, while knowing sets the stage, it is through action that one truly engages with and influences the world.

REFERENCES

Holme JA, Refsnes M, Dybing E. Mulig kreftrisiko ved tilvirkning og bruk av kreosotimpregnert trevirke [Possible carcinogenic risk associated with production and use of creosote-treated wood]. Tidsskr Nor Laegeforen. 1999 Aug 10;119(18):2664-6. Norwegian. PMID: 10479980.

IARC (International Agency for Research on Cancer). (1999). *IARC Monographs on the Evaluation of Carcinogenic Risks to Humans: Volume 72*. World Health Organization.

IARC (International Agency for Research on Cancer). (2006). *IARC Monographs on the Evaluation of Carcinogenic Risks to Humans: Volume 86*. World Health Organization.

IARC Working Group on the Evaluation of Carcinogenic Risks to Humans. Some Industrial Chemicals. Lyon (FR): International Agency for Research on Cancer; 2000. (IARC Monographs on the Evaluation of Carcinogenic Risks to Humans, No. 77.) Ethylbenzene.

International Agency for Research on Cancer (IARC). (1980). *IARC Monographs on the Evaluation of the Carcinogenic Risk of Chemicals to Humans: Volume 22*. (p. 55). World Health Organization.

International Agency for Research on Cancer. (2015). *IARC Monograph on Glyphosate*. Lyon, France: International Agency for Research on Cancer. Retrieved from https://www.iarc.who.int/featured-news/media-centre-iarc-news-glyphosate/

Unraveling the Origins: Exploring 101 Triggers of Cancer

National Cancer Institute CARCINOGENESIS. Technical Report Series 186, U.S. Department of Health, Education and Welfare, Public Health Services, National Institute of Health, 1979.

National Cancer Institute. (2017). *NCI Technical Report Series No. 24*. U.S. Department of Health and Human Services, National Institutes of Health. Retrieved from https://www.ncbi.nlm.nih.gov/pmc/articles/PMC7905528/

NCIC (National Chemical Information Center). (1979). *NCIC No. 191, CAS No. 108-60-1*.

National Institutes of Health, Department of Health and Human Services, NTPTOX1, Publication No. 91-3120 (1991)

National Toxicology Program, 1995, National Toxicology Program Technical Report Series, ISSN: *0888-8051*,
U.S. Department of Health, Public Health Service, National Institutes of Health

National Toxicology Program. Report on Carcinogens, 1st Edition. U.S. Department of Health and Human Services, Public Health Service, National Toxicology Program, 1980.

National Toxicology Program. Technology Report 499, Indium Phosphide, (CAS NO. 22398-80-7) IN F344/N RATS AND B6C3F1 MICE (Inhalation Studies) 2001.

National Library of Medicine. (2012). Genotoxicity of food preservative sodium sorbate in human lymphocytes in vitro. PubMed Central.

National Toxicology Program. Report on Carcinogens, 2nd Edition. U.S. Department of Health and Human Services, Public Health Service, National Toxicology Program, 1981.

National Toxicology Program. Report on Carcinogens, 3rd Edition. U.S. Department of Health and Human Services, Public Health Service, National Toxicology Program, 1982.

National Toxicology Program. Report on Carcinogens, 4th Edition. U.S. Department of Health and Human Services, Public Health Service, National Toxicology Program, 1985.

National Toxicology Program. Report on Carcinogens, 5th Edition. U.S. Department of Health and Human Services, Public Health Service, National Toxicology Program, 1989.

National Toxicology Program. Report on Carcinogens, 6th Edition. U.S. Department of Health and Human Services, Public Health Service, National Toxicology Program, 1991.

National Toxicology Program. Report on Carcinogens, 7th Edition. U.S. Department of Health and Human Services, Public Health Service, National Toxicology Program, 1994.

National Toxicology Program. Report on Carcinogens, 8th Edition. U.S. Department of Health and Human Services, Public Health Service, National Toxicology Program, 1998.

National Toxicology Program. Report on Carcinogens, 9th Edition. U.S. Department of Health and Human Services, Public Health Service, National Toxicology Program, 2000.

National Toxicology Program. Report on Carcinogens, 10th Edition. U.S. Department of Health and Human Services, Public Health Service, National Toxicology Program, 2002.

National Toxicology Program. Report on Carcinogens, 11th Edition. U.S. Department of Health and Human Services, Public Health Service, National Toxicology Program, 2005.

National Toxicology Program. Report on Carcinogens, 12th Edition. U.S. Department of Health and Human Services, Public Health Service, National Toxicology Program, 2011.

National Toxicology Program. Report on Carcinogens, 13th Edition. U.S. Department of Health and Human Services, Public Health Service, National Toxicology Program, 2014.

National Toxicology Program. Report on Carcinogens, 14th Edition. U.S. Department of Health and Human Services, Public Health Service, National Toxicology Program, 2016.

National Toxicology Program. Report on Carcinogens, 15th Edition. U.S. Department of Health and Human Services, Public Health Service, National Toxicology Program, 2019.

National Toxicology Program. (2017). *Antimony Trioxide*. Technical Report 590.

NTP. Etoposide (33419-42-0). Chemical Effects in Biological Systems (CEBS). Research Triangle Park, NC (USA): National Toxicology Program (NTP). Accessed 2024-07-04.

NTP; TOXICOLOGY AND CARCINOGENESIS STUDIES OF N,N-DIMETHYL-p-TOLUIDINE (CAS NO. 99-97-8) IN F344/N RATS AND B6C3F1/N MICE (GAVAGE STUDIES) NTP TR 579 NIH Publication No. 12-5921 (September 2012)

Radoï L, Sylla F, Matrat M, Barul C, Menvielle G, Delafosse P, Stücker I, Luce D; ICARE study group. Head and neck cancer and occupational exposure to leather dust: results from the ICARE study, a French case-control study. Environ Health. 2019 Mar 29;18(1):27. doi: 10.1186/s12940-019-0469-3. PMID: 30922305; PMCID: PMC6440008.

Salerno M, Cascio O, Bertozzi G, Sessa F, Messina A, Monda V, Cipolloni L, Biondi A, Daniele A, Pomara C. Anabolic androgenic steroids and carcinogenicity focusing on Leydig cell: a literature review. Oncotarget. 2018 Apr 10;9(27):19415-19426. doi: 10.18632/oncotarget.24767. PMID: 29721213; PMCID: PMC5922407.

SEER Cancer Statistics Factsheets: Common Cancer Sites. National Cancer Institute. Bethesda, MD.

Siegel RL, Giaquinto, AN, Jemal A. Cancer statistics, 2024. *CA: A Cancer Journal for Clinicians* 2024; 74(1):1–114.

U.S. Environmental Protection Agency. (2021, August). *Toxicological Review of tert-Butyl Alcohol (tert-Butanol) [CASRN 75-65-0]*.

INDEX

adrenal, 77, 79, 228
agriculture, 113, 115, 129, 162, 207, 208, 216, 248, 251, 256, 258
alcohol, 30, 31, 35, 59, 60, 68, 93
alkylating, 108, 130, 135, 136, 162, 198, 225, 232, 253
biological, 14, 21, 22, 26, 58, 65, 67, 69, 73, 117, 164, 165, 193, 233, 247, 281

bladder, 8, 44, 45, 75, 76, 83, 95, 96, 99, 103, 104, 105, 111, 112, 114, 117, 119, 149, 155, 156, 158, 200, 201, 207, 218, 232, 253
Blood, 12, 71
brain, 47, 61, 63, 81, 83, 108, 110, 135, 136, 169, 259, 270
breast, 53, 57, 59, 60, 81, 85, 88, 90, 92, 99, 101, 102, 106, 107, 144, 145, 146, 147, 148, 169, 183, 232, 238, 242, 243, 253
cervical, 65, 66, 148
chemical, 21, 26, 27, 36, 42, 43, 44, 45, 47, 51, 53, 59, 61, 63, 75, 79, 81, 82, 83, 85, 90, 94, 96, 97, 98, 101, 103, 105, 108, 109, 113, 117, 119, 120, 121, 123, 125, 126, 127, 128, 130, 131, 135, 138, 139, 140, 141, 144, 147, 149, 152, 155, 159, 161, 162, 163, 164, 167, 168, 170, 171, 172, 173, 176, 177, 178, 179, 180, 181, 182, 183, 184, 186, 188, 191, 192, 195, 198, 200, 202, 204, 205, 207, 210, 213, 216, 218, 219, 220, 221, 223, 224, 226, 228, 231, 234, 236, 238, 240, 242, 244, 245, 246, 248, 250, 251, 253, 255, 256, 257, 259, 260, 261, 263, 267, 270, 273
Chemical, 14
chemotherapy, 8, 9, 10, 13, 18, 27, 107, 108, 109, 130, 131, 135, 136, 184, 185, 186, 198, 204, 205, 224, 225, 232, 253
Chemotherapy, 4
colon, 61, 73, 83, 164, 165, 188, 221, 226
endometrial, 101, 102, 106, 107, 144, 145, 146, 147, 239
environment, 23, 41, 43, 47, 54, 58, 70, 77, 78, 80, 86, 93, 113, 114, 115, 116,

255

125, 127, 129, 133, 138, 139, 141, 149, 151, 162, 164, 174, 181, 183, 187, 192, 197, 202, 203, 208, 209, 211, 213, 214, 217, 236, 237, 249, 251, 252, 258, 264, 273
environmental, 192, 202, 211, 214, 217, 229, 237, 252, 282
Environmental, 14, 22, 52, 97, 127, 141, 164, 166, 183
eye, 55, 206, 223, 248, 261
FDA, 10, 33, 34, 38, 64, 111, 160, 226
fungicides, 113, 115, 161, 247
herbicides, 54, 113, 115, 161, 187, 202, 221, 237, 247, 258, 266
herbs, 10, 66, 69
humors, 11, 12
inflammation, 15, 66, 68, 70, 71, 73, 74, 93, 110, 112, 122, 143, 154, 158, 190, 244, 273
insecticides, 113, 115, 161, 247
kidney, 51, 52, 75, 83, 94, 95, 96, 109, 111, 112, 149, 163, 173, 186, 207, 228, 237, 264
larynx, 50, 59
leukemia, 47, 49, 57, 77, 79, 82, 88, 108, 109, 113, 127, 130, 131, 135, 137, 141, 182, 183, 184, 185, 186, 202, 204, 223, 224, 226, 228, 231, 240, 251, 253, 256, 264, 265
liver, 51, 52, 53, 59, 61, 63, 64, 67, 68, 73, 74, 75, 77, 79, 83, 91, 93, 104, 109, 114, 119, 128, 131, 133, 134, 138, 163, 181, 187, 191, 202, 203, 207, 216, 217, 218, 227, 228, 236, 237, 239, 240, 241, 244, 245, 246, 248, 252, 255, 257, 259, 260, 264, 265, 268, 270
lung, 7, 36, 40, 44, 45, 49, 50, 53, 57, 61, 63, 64, 77, 79, 80, 81, 83, 85, 88, 89, 96, 99, 113, 114, 119, 121, 122, 125, 126, 135, 138, 140, 141, 143, 144, 149, 152, 154, 179, 180, 184, 188, 190, 192, 196, 198, 204, 205, 206, 207, 213, 214, 234, 244, 260, 264, 272
lymphatic, 63, 198, 207, 265
lymphoma, 53, 69, 70, 77, 79, 82, 108, 113, 127, 130, 135, 138, 141, 182, 183, 184, 185, 204, 225, 251, 253, 255, 258, 261, 262
meat, 55, 120, 230
mesothelioma, 38, 49, 50, 125, 179, 180

Unraveling the Origins: Exploring 101 Triggers of Cancer

mouth, 44, 45, 59, 193
mutations, 8, 13, 27, 28, 55, 58, 59, 66, 70, 73, 76, 94, 101, 104, 108, 109, 118, 119, 122, 127, 129, 134, 136, 137, 141, 155, 158, 162, 182, 185, 201, 207, 217, 227, 233, 262, 269
nasal, 47, 80, 99, 161, 167, 173, 176, 213, 220
National Toxicology Program, 15, 21, 127, 205, 278, 279, 280, 281
nose, 49, 170
oil, 126, 210, 265, 267, 272, 273
oral, 25, 31, 65, 93, 123, 124, 167, 239
ovarian, 38, 50, 106, 130, 144, 146, 198, 239, 253
PAHs, 44, 85, 86, 87, 97, 99, 120, 150, 211, 272
pancreas, 73, 149, 236
pharmaceutical, 27, 30, 33, 104, 139, 161, 175, 176, 192, 232, 246
pharynx, 50, 59, 123
physical, 14, 272
prostate, 16, 53, 90, 92, 93, 149, 242
radiation, 3, 57, 58
rectum, 149
resin, 63, 172, 177
Resins, 48, 172, 220
sarcoma, 53, 193, 194, 225, 261

skin, 31, 39, 53, 55, 56, 58, 62, 64, 65, 80, 85, 91, 97, 114, 119, 125, 127, 138, 140, 150, 161, 171, 175, 176, 181, 183, 193, 194, 198, 201, 203, 204, 206, 207, 210, 211, 212, 214, 215, 221, 235, 236, 244, 245, 248, 255, 257, 261, 262, 264, 265
stomach, 50, 61, 62, 69, 70, 71, 72, 83, 85, 113, 119, 170, 176, 198, 232, 263, 267
synthetic, 26, 27, 30, 75, 90, 106, 107, 110, 111, 117, 126, 127, 128, 132, 139, 159, 160, 181, 186, 191, 192, 218, 219, 220, 224, 233, 236, 238, 239, 240, 265, 266, 268, 274
testicular, 77, 79, 90, 159, 161, 185, 241
throat, 44, 45, 49, 50, 66, 72
thyroid, 29, 30, 31, 32, 57, 88, 128, 129, 131, 170, 200, 216, 217, 268
tobacco, 13, 14, 28, 35, 36, 37, 44, 45, 46, 61, 62, 78, 87, 93, 99, 100, 119, 123, 124, 228, 264, 266
uterus, 81, 101, 102, 107, 146, 147, 259
virus, 66, 67, 68, 69, 74, 193, 194, 262

World Health Organization,
 17, 32, 56, 150, 235, 256,
 258, 277

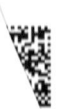
www.ingramcontent.com/pod-product-compliance
Lightning Source LLC
Chambersburg PA
CBHW041038050426
42337CB00058B/4910